Patient-Centered Care Series

Series Editors

Moira Stewart,
Judith Belle Brown
and
Thomas R Freeman

Substance Abuse

A patient-centered approach

Edited by
Michael R Floyd
and
J Paul Seale

Radcliffe Medical Press

Radcliffe Medical Press Ltd
18 Marcham Road
Abingdon
Oxon OX14 1AA
United Kingdom

www.radcliffe-oxford.com
The Radcliffe Medical Press electronic catalogue and online ordering facility.
Direct sales to anywhere in the world.

British Library Cataloguing in Publication Data

A catalogue record for this book is available from the British Library.

ISBN 1 85775 912 5

Typeset by Aarontype Ltd, Easton, Bristol
Printed and bound by TJ International Ltd, Padstow, Cornwall

Contents

Series editors' introduction

The strength of medicine in curing many infectious diseases and some of the chronic diseases has also led to a key weakness. Some believe that medicine has abdicated its caring role and, in doing so, has not only alienated the public to some extent, but also failed to uphold its promise to 'do no harm'. One hears many stories of patients who have been technically cured but feel ill or who feel ill but for whom no satisfactory diagnosis is possible. In focusing so much attention on the nature of the disease, medicine has neglected the person who suffers the disease. Redressing this 20th century phenomenon required a new definition of medicine's role for the 21st century. A new clinical method, which has been developed during the 1980s and 1990s, has attempted to correct the flaw, to regain the balance between curing and caring. It is the called patient-centered clinical method and has been described and illustrated in *Patient-Centered Medicine: Transforming the Clinical Method* (Stewart *et al.*, 1995) of which the 2nd edition is being prepared for publication in early 2003. In the 1995 book, conceptual, educational and research issues were elucidated in detail. The patient-centered conceptual framework from that book is used as the structure for each book in the series introduced here; it consists of six interactive components to be considered in every patient–practitioner interaction.

The first component is to assess the two modes of ill health: disease and illness. In addition to assessing the disease process, the clinician explores the patient's illness experience. Specifically, the practitioner considers how the patient feels about being ill, what the patient's ideas are about the illness, what impact the illness is having on the patient's functioning and what he or she expects from the clinician.

The second component is an integration of the concepts of disease and illness with an understanding of the whole person. This includes an awareness of the patient's position in the lifecycle and the social context in which they live.

The third component of the method is the mutual task of finding common ground between the patient and the practitioner. This consists of three key areas: mutually defining the problem, mutually defining the goals of management/treatment, and mutually exploring the roles to be assumed by the patient and the practitioner.

The fourth component is to use each visit as an opportunity for prevention and health promotion. The fifth component takes into consideration that each encounter with the patient should be used to develop the helping relationship;

the trust and respect that evolve in the relationship will have an impact on other components of the method. The sixth component requires that, throughout the process, the practitioner is realistic in terms of time, availability of resources and the amount of emotional and physical energy needed.

However, there is a gap between the description of the clinical method and its application in practice. The series of books presented here attempts to bridge that gap. Written by international leaders in their field, the series represents clinical explications of the patient-centered clinical method. Each volume deals with a common and challenging problem faced by practitioners. In each book, current thinking is organized in a similar way, reinforcing and illustrating the patient-centered clinical method. The common format begins with a description of the burden of illness, followed by chapters on the illness experience, the disease, the whole person, the patient–practitioner relationship and finding common ground, including current therapeutics.

The book series is international, contributors to date representing Norway, Canada, Australia, New Zealand and the USA. This is a testament to the universality of the values and concepts inherent in the patient-centered clinical method. The work of not only the authors but others who have studied patients has reinforced a virtually identical series of six components (Little *et al.*, 2001; Stewart, 2001). We feel that there is an emerging international definition of patient-centered practice which is represented in this book series.

The vigor of any clinical method is proven in the extent to which it is applicable in the clinical setting. It is anticipated that this series will inform further development of the clinical method and move thinking forward in this important aspect of medicine.

Moira Stewart PhD
Judith Belle Brown PhD
Thomas R Freeman MD, CCFP

About the authors

Sonya Cashdan PhD is Associate Professor of English at East Tennessee State University, where she has taught courses about medicine in literature as well as women's studies. Her research interests include female heroes and medical ethics. She has published articles for the National Endowment for the Humanities and is at present writing two entries for Magill's *Medical Guide: Pediatrics*.

Jerome D Cook PhD is a clinical psychologist, certified by the APA College of Professional Psychology in the Treatment of Alcohol and Other Psychoactive Substance Use Disorders. His clinical practice is with the Substance Abuse Treatment Program, James H Quillen Veterans Affairs Medical Center, and he holds a clinical appointment with the Department of Psychiatry at the James H Quillen College of Medicine.

Michael R Floyd EdD is a licensed psychologist and Associate Professor of Family Medicine at the James H Quillen College of Medicine, East Tennessee State University, certified by the APA College of Professional Psychology in the Treatment of Alcohol and Other Psychoactive Substance Use Disorders. Along with colleagues at East Tennessee State University, he has conducted national and international workshops, lectured and written numerous articles in the area of doctor–patient communication. He has experience in treating substance use disorders in both inpatient and outpatient settings. He has chaired the Tennessee Psychological Association Colleague Assistance program and written articles in the area of professional impairment and substance abuse.

Antonnette V Graham PhD, LISW, RN is Professor of Family Medicine, General Medical Science (Adolescent Health) and Nursing at Case Western Reserve University. During her 20 years in family medicine she has chaired the STFM Working Group on Substance Abuse, served as treasurer of the Association for Medical Education and Research in Substance Abuse, and developed curricula on substance abuse for medical students, residents and continuing medical education programs. Her writings on substance abuse have appeared in social science and medical journals and textbooks, and she has lectured on this topic in the US, Europe and Asia.

Ronald S McCord MS, MD, MClSc, AAFP died unexpectedly during the preparation of this book. He was a family physician and Associate Professor of Family Medicine at the James H Quillen College of Medicine, East Tennessee State University. Along with colleagues at East Tennessee State University, he conducted national and international workshops, lectured and wrote numerous articles in the area of doctor–patient communication. Dr McCord completed a fellowship in academic family medicine at the University of Western Ontario, and taught patient-centered medicine at the University of Arkansas for Medical Sciences and the University of Illinois College of Medicine at Rockford, Illinois.

Myra Muramoto MD is a family physician and Assistant Professor of Family and Community Medicine, University of Arizona College of Medicine, Tucson, Arizona. Dr Muramoto is active in both substance abuse education (for local, state, national and international projects) and substance abuse research, where she has conducted public health and clinical trial research on substance abuse problems. Her clinical experience with this population includes inpatient settings, as well as primary care-based prevention and outpatient treatment.

Gregory Phelps MD, MPH is a family physician and Medical Director of St Mary's Occupational Health Services, Knoxville, Tennessee. He is certified by the American Board of Family Practice, Occupational Medicine, and the American Society of Addiction Medicine. He has served as medical director for two ambulatory addiction treatment facilities and taught substance abuse as Associate Professor at Mercer University School of Medicine, Macon, Georgia, where he published four book chapters and 20 scholarly articles.

Jerome Schulz MD, FAAFP is a family physician and Associate Clinical Professor at East Carolina University School of Medicine, Greenville, North Carolina, where he is a consultant for addiction. Certified by the American Society of Addiction Medicine, Dr Schulz has written over 15 articles and book chapters pertaining to drug/alcohol addiction problems in patients. He has been a member of two STFM national contracts with the Center for Substance Abuse Prevention and the National Institute for Alcoholism and Alcohol Abuse, to develop curricula in the field of drug/alcohol addiction and prevention.

J Paul Seale MD, FAAFP is a family physician and Associate Professor of Family and Community Medicine at the Mercer University School of Medicine and the Medical Center of Central Georgia in Macon, Georgia. He completed a fellowship in Substance Abuse Teaching in Family Medicine sponsored by STFM, the National Institute on Alcohol Abuse and Alcoholism and the National Institute for Drug Abuse. He has been involved in substance abuse education at the University of Texas Health Science Center, San Antonio, Texas, and the University of Zulia in Maracaibo, Venezuela. He has also been involved in substance abuse research with Hispanic, African American and Native American populations. Dr Seale is a member of the American Society of Addiction Medicine (ASAM).

Sylvia Shellenberger PhD is Professor of Family and Community Medicine at Mercer University School of Medicine, and Director of Psychology and Education in the Department of Family Medicine, where she teaches family medicine residents how to create and maintain a positive doctor–patient relationship whilst managing patients' psychological and substance abuse issues. She specializes in family and couples work, including those in recovery from substance abuse. The author of numerous chapters and journal articles, she also serves on numerous editorial boards, including *Professional Psychology* and *Families, Systems and Health*.

James Turnbull MD PhD is a psychiatrist and Medical Director for Outpatient Services at Frontier Health Inc, where he treats substance-abusing patients. He is Clinical Professor of Psychiatry and Family Medicine at the James H Quillen College of Medicine, East Tennessee State University, and has been an examiner for the American Board of Psychiatry and Neurology. He has published over 50 articles and several book chapters.

Jack R Woodside Jr MD is Associate Director of the Johnson City Family Practice Residency Program and Associate Professor of Family Medicine at the James H Quillen College of Medicine, East Tennessee State University, where he assumes responsibility for curriculum development and teaching on substance use disorders for medical students, residents and continuing medical education programs. Dr Woodside is certified by the American Board of Family Practice and the American Society of Addiction Medicine. He has treated substance-abusing patients in both inpatient and primary care settings, and is the Regional Director of the Tennessee Medical Association Physicians' Health Program, Recovery Aftercare Monitoring Rehabilitation team.

Acknowledgments

Along the way toward completion of this project we lost a friend, collaborator and colleague through an untimely death, Ronald McCord MD. His meritorious work deserves special recognition and his ideas will be missed.

We would like to acknowledge the support of our respective academic institutions: East Tennessee State University, James H Quillen College of Medicine in Johnson City, Tennessee, Mercer University School of Medicine and the Medical Center of Central Georgia in Macon, Georgia. For encouragement and reallocation of work duties, we extend our thanks to Jim Wilson MD and TW Treadwell Jr MD, Chairs of our Departments of Family Medicine, and Elizabeth McCord MD and Fred Girton MD, Program Directors of our Family Practice Residency Programs.

Completing a project such as this requires the efforts of many individuals. We are grateful for the encouragement and critical thinking offered by colleagues within our Departments of Family Medicine and Family Practice Residency Programs. I (MRF) would like to express special appreciation to the colleagues of the East Tennessee State University Interview Study Group: Drs Kathleen Beine, Elizabeth McCord and Patricia Buck for their friendship, creative energy, valuable insights and editorial assistance; to Carol Abel and Ruth Albrecht for years of technical assistance; and to Phyllis Livesay, Dixie Stanton-Matayka, and Alice Johnson for manuscript preparation. Lastly, and most significantly, heartfelt thanks to Forrest Lang, MD, for his mentoring, personal attention, innovative thinking, perseverance and leadership through the Interview Study Group.

Finally, we thank our patients and clients who have had courage to share with us about themselves, and in so doing have taught us most of what we have communicated in this book.

Dedication

To my wife Dana, who fills my life with joy, light and her incredible insights into human behavior and true spirituality; and to my children, Josiah, Julie, Jonathan and Jenni, who have taught me how to love, play, encourage and to keep pressing forward. – JPS

To my parents, Joseph E and Jeanne M Floyd, wife Susanna, and children, Anna and Benjamin, for their constant love, encouragement and support. – MRF

Introduction

Ronald S McCord and Michael R Floyd

Substance use disorders

Drug and alcohol addiction is a leading cause of rising healthcare costs. Drug and alcohol addiction cost the US $70 billion each year in medical costs, legal problems and lost time at work. Drug and alcohol problems double the healthcare costs for patients (Holder, 1987). With an increasing emphasis on managed care, the need for primary care physicians to improve their detection and to intervene in drug and alcohol problems is urgent.

Although physicians naturally believe they are patient-centered because they are trying to help their patients, the concept of a patient-centered clinical method refers to a specific clinical approach that involves much more than just diagnosing and treating disease. The patient-centered clinical method evolved from developments in other disciplines, including the contributions of Carl Rogers, a psychologist who developed client-centered psychotherapy (1958). During the decades of the 1970s and 1980s, significant thought was being given to the patients' perspective by a number of authors in the discipline of family medicine; for example, Ian McWhinney (1972), Gayle Stephens (1982), Lynn Carmichael (1985) and Joseph Levenstein (1984). In the early 1980s, Levenstein (1984) brought his concepts of a patient-centered clinical method to the University of Western Ontario (Carmichael, 1985).

Early identification and intervention has been demonstrated to be effective in reducing the rates and consequences of substance abuse, yet clinicians do not always address this issue (Burge and Schneider, 1999; Fleming, 1993; Fleming *et al.*, 1997, 1998). Often neither the patient nor the clinician is aware of or, indeed, wants to engage in what are expected to be difficult problems.

A detailed discussion of causes and theories associated with substance abuse and addiction goes well beyond the scope of this volume. A wide range of biopsychosocial factors is thought to contribute to the development and maintenance of substance use disorders (Marlatt and VandenBos, 1997). Biological factors include genetic predisposition, associated inherited traits leading to increased vulnerability to substance abuse or problematic mood states. Social and cultural issues also play a major role in the types of drugs to which individuals are introduced. Psychological factors include classical and operant conditioning, social learning theory (Bandura, 1977) and cognitive psychology (Beck, 1976; Beck *et al.*, 1993; Ellis *et al.*, 1988). Other important theorists include Zimberg *et al.* (1987), Blane and Leonard (1987), and Leeds and Morgenstern (1996). Several family theory models provide a framework for understanding substance use disorders. These include family systems, family disease models and behavioral/learning theory (Margolis and Zweben, 1998).

Recently, expectancy theorists (Blane and Leonard, 1987; Leonard and Blane, 1999), cognitive behavioral psychologists (Beck *et al.*, 1993) and behaviorists have provided useful models explaining health-related behavior and offered practical, patient-centered approaches for addressing substance use concerns with patients (Miller and Heather, 1998; Prochaska and DiClemente, 1986; Prochaska *et al.*, 1992; Rollnick *et al.*, 1992, 1999).

The National Institute on Drug Abuser's (NIDA) 13 principles of effective drug treatment (Leshner, 2000) give strong support for a patient-centered approach for helping substance abusers. The first principle is, 'No single treatment is appropriate for all individuals'. Principle Three states that effective treatment attends to 'multiple needs of the individual, not just his or her drug use' and Principle Four states, '. . . [the] plan must be assessed continually and modified as necessary to assure that the plan meets the person's changing needs'.

It is not the purpose of this book to solve the controversial 'disease' vs 'learning' model debate. However, it is important for clinicians to be aware of these models and of their implications for treatment. Recognizing that as much as 93% of addictive treatment in the US is 12-step abstinence based (Horvath, 2000), many of our recommendations, especially for the small percentage of the alcohol and drug-abusing population that is chemically dependent, are for abstinence. This is not to say that other methods would not be helpful. Several other important treatment models need to be considered by patients and clinicians. These methods include Rational Recovery (RR), Women for Sobriety (WFS), Self-Management and Recovery Training (SMART), and harm reduction approaches (Denning, 2000a, b; Donovan, 1998; Weingardt and Marlatt, 1998).

Clinicians' beliefs and expectations of disease and treatment outcomes, as well as biasing and stereotyping, affect communication with persons who might have substance use disorders. Patients and their families also maintain a set of values and expectations, rooted in history and community lore as well as in past experience with the disease process and with health providers themselves.

Clinicians bring a unique personal history regarding the use of mood-altering chemicals into the clinical setting that can profoundly influence clinical judgment and practice. Negative attitudes toward substance abusers may result from past experiences with difficult patients, negative role models, inadequate education and skills training, overexposure to chronic (relapsing) patients, lack of exposure to successfully recovering patients, lack of accessible treatment facilities and concerns about the clinician's own substance abuse (Seale, 1991). As students and clinicians acquire a more comprehensive understanding of substance use disorders and learn more effective methods for addressing these problems, they will appreciate successes that will be self-reinforcing. This will come about as their preceptors and teachers demonstrate successful methods for communicating both non-judgmental expressions of their own concerns for patient welfare as well as an understanding of the patient's concerns. Negative attitudes about substance-abusing patients will change when teachers demonstrate ways of accepting and working with these individuals rather than as someone to be ignored or 'turfed'. As teachers model effective ways of communicating, negotiating and motivating behavior change, learners will more appropriately assess and treat substance-abusing patients.

It is our hope that readers of this volume will recognize the utility of combining an understanding of substance use disorders with the methods and philosophy of the patient-centered approach.

Magnitude of the problem: painting the mosaic of substance abuse in a multiethnic society

J Paul Seale and Myra Muramoto

Editor's introduction

The first component of the patient-centered model, demonstrated and described for the first time by Levenstein in the 1980s (1984), involves exploring both the disease and the patient's illness experience. The first step in this process is to understand the specific disease in question. Brown et al. (1995) describe 'disease' as medical science's abstract description of what is wrong with the body as a machine. There are few diseases where genetic and sociocultural factors result in such a wide variation in disease presentation as in the disease of substance abuse. For example, the differences in presentation between an adolescent Native American male who presents with neutropenia from repeated experimentation with inhalants and an 80-year-old Caucasian socialite who suffers a fractured hip due to dizziness caused by her chronic benzodiazepine abuse is so marked as to appear to be two entirely different diseases. Upon closer examination, nonetheless, we find that both patients demonstrate the pattern of continuing use of psychoactive substances despite adverse consequences, which is the hallmark of this disease. In Chapter 1, we will focus primarily on the epidemiologic patterns of disease presentation of substance abuse as it spans the gamut of age, gender and ethnic background. Later, in Chapter 2, we will give greater attention to the illness experience of those affected by this disease, which represents the 'other half' of the first component of patient-centered medicine.

Case study

Bobby M is a 52-year-old peanut farmer referred to the regional trauma center from a rural South Georgia hospital for management of a compound lower extremity fracture following a motor vehicle accident. His past medical history is unremarkable. Bobby is divorced, lives alone and admits to drinking 'only three or four beers per day, mostly on the weekends'. On the second hospital day he becomes slightly tremulous and anxious with mild elevation of his pulse and blood pressure. The physician is stopped in the hall by the patient's sister Wilma, who expresses concern regarding his substance use. She explains that Bobby was previously employed as a school bus driver, but lost his job some three years ago due to a positive urine drug screen for marijuana. Since his divorce, Wilma reports that Bobby has become more and more regular in stopping by the bar two miles down the highway from his peanut farm after work each day. She is concerned because he drives his pickup truck home around midnight most evenings after 'having a few cold ones' with his friends. She has invited him to attend an Alcoholics Anonymous meeting where she is a regular attender, but thus far he has refused. She is eager for his physician to try to 'get through to him' before something more serious happens.

Substance abuse is a multifaceted illness, which manifests itself in radically different ways among different segments of North America's culturally diverse population. While the casual or 'social' use of mood-altering substances such as alcohol, tobacco or marijuana is common in many societies, use of increasing amounts of such substances and more frequent use can cause significant negative consequences in a variety of life areas. Individuals move, often silently and insidiously, from low-risk use to at-risk use and eventually into problematic use which places their own health and that of their families in danger (*see* Figure 1.1). Individuals may progress to a point where use of alcohol, marijuana, heroin, cocaine or other psychoactive substances results in repeated

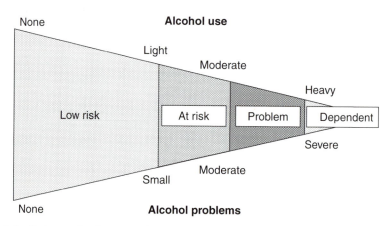

Figure 1.1 Relationship between alcohol use and alcohol problems (NIAAA, 1998).

adverse health, job, family, legal or other consequences affecting both themselves and those around them – a syndrome called 'alcohol or drug abuse'. A key hallmark of the abuse syndrome is continuing use of psychoactive substances in spite of such adverse consequences, a cycle of events which results in mounting harm to patients, their families, their employers and their communities. Many patients affected by psychoactive substance abuse at some time in their lives also experience alcohol or drug dependency. This is a more serious disorder characterized by compulsive use of alcohol or drugs and loss of control over the amount consumed. Two important characteristics of the dependency syndrome include the development over time of physiologic tolerance (the necessity to consume greater and greater amounts of the psychoactive substance in order to produce the same affective response) and the emergence of withdrawal symptoms when substance use is interrupted for any reason. The natural course of alcohol- and drug-related disorder is unpredictable, at times marked by a rapid downhill course, at other times interspersed with repeated remissions and in other cases ending in full recovery after only a short period of time (Vaillant, 1995). In this book, we will utilize the term 'substance abuse' to refer to repetitive problematic use of alcohol or other psychoactive drugs, with or without the development of a dependency syndrome. It is the burden of this clinical syndrome that we will attempt to summarize in this chapter.

While alcohol remains the primary drug of abuse in most societies, over the past decade the combined use of both alcohol and other drugs has become increasingly commonplace in many parts of the world. Substance abuse is costly to society, as well as to the individuals it affects. Drug and alcohol addiction cost the US $70 billion each year in medical costs, legal problems and lost time at work. Drug and alcohol problems are also a leading cause of rising healthcare costs, with studies indicating a doubling of healthcare costs for affected patients (Holder, 1987). Continuing research among a variety of ethnic populations has revealed significant variations in the prevalence and presentation of substance abuse disorders, depending on the gender, age and ethnic background of the population. Earlier research findings, based primarily on studies of Caucasian male patients, may not be representative of the experience of women or of patients from other ethnic backgrounds. While there are widely held beliefs that alcohol and drug problems are more prevalent among social/ethnic minorities, and that morbidity and mortality related to these disorders are more serious in minorities, these generalizations are not always supported by scientific data.

In this chapter we will review data from formal surveys such as the Epidemiological Catchment Area (ECA) study, the Hispanic Health and Nutrition Examination Survey (Hispanic HANES), and recent primary care intervention trials as well as several qualitative studies, in an attempt to paint the mosaic of the substance abuse as it cuts across boundaries of gender and ethnicity in North America. We will look in some detail at the presentation of substance abuse problems among four major North American ethnic groups: Whites, African Americans, Hispanic Americans, and Native Americans. We will then describe recently developed definitions of at-risk drinking patterns, which may be used by clinicians to identify patients who may benefit from risk reduction interventions.

Current population profile

Available data on alcohol use in the general US population come primarily from national surveys performed on household populations which exclude institutionalized and homeless persons. Questions include quantity and frequency of alcohol consumption and consequences of alcohol use. Examples are the 1983 and 1988 National Health Interview Surveys (NHISs), the smaller 1984 and 1990 National Alcohol Surveys (NASs) and National Household Health Survey (NHHS) (USDHHS, 1991), and the Alcohol Research Group's (ARG) 1984 and 1992 surveys of a national multiethnic sample (Caetano, 1997). In addition, studies such as the ECA study from the early 1980s (Regier *et al.*, 1990) and the National Longitudinal Study of Youth (NLSY; Harford and Grant, 1994) measure the prevalence of alcohol and drug abuse or dependency using diagnostic criteria from *Diagnostic and Statistical Manual*, 3rd edition (DSM III) or its revision (DSM III-R). The ECA study was a one-time sampling of households in five population centers in different parts of the US while the NLSY is a cohort study of 12 000 men and women aged between 14 and 21 in January of 1979 who were interviewed in 1979 and again in 1989. The Hispanic HANES surveyed patterns of abstention and frequent heavy drinking among 7471 Mexican Americans, Puerto Ricans, and Cuban Americans between 1982 and 1984. To date, however, there has been no comprehensive federal effort to collect alcohol or drug abuse information on Native American/ Alaskan Native populations. As a result, much of the alcohol and drug use data on Native American and Alaskan Natives come from on-going school-based surveys on American Indian youth conducted by the Tri-ethnic Center for Prevention Research at Colorado State University, and from regional, state and local studies. From these studies, we gain the following perspective on the burden of alcohol and drug problems in the United States.

In the current US population, two-thirds of adults consume alcohol, and 34.6% also report psychoactive drug use at some point in their lives (USDHHS, 1997, 1998). Men report higher rates of use of most psychoactive substances. More men than women drink, drink 'heavily,' and experience alcohol use-related problems. Alcohol dependency is two–three times as prevalent in men as in women in the US (Grant, 1997b). Men are also more likely to use most illicit drugs, and use of marijuana and cocaine, the most commonly used drugs, is substantially greater in men than women (Johnston *et al.* 1993; USDHHS, 1998). Multiple drug use appears to be increasingly common, especially among cohorts 18–34 years old (USDHHS, 1993). Concurrent use of alcohol and illicit drugs appears to be increasing among women, especially at younger ages (Lex, 1991). Some trends in alcohol use in the US are encouraging. *Per capita* alcohol use in the US has been declining since 1981, after some 50 years of gradual increase (Midanik and Clark, 1994; USDHHS, 1997). Analysis of various age cohorts reveals highest rates of alcohol abuse and dependency among young White males, with several studies indicating that alcohol use and heavy drinking in this age group are slowly decreasing (Caetano and Clark, 1998).

Women

Although not all authors agree, many investigators are convinced that the gap between male and female substance abuse is narrowing (Hughes *et al.*, 1997; Mercer and Kavari, 1990; Wilsnack and Wilsnack, 1995). Teenage girls (aged 12–17) interviewed as part of the 1997 National Household Survey on Drug Abuse (NHSDA) were as or more likely than teenage boys to have used alcohol, cigarettes, cocaine, crack, sedatives, tranquilizers, analgesics, hallucinogens and inhalants in the past year (USDHHS, 1998). Midanik and Clark, in their analysis of changes in drinking patterns of adults between 1984–90, found declines on six different measures of alcohol use in men between 1984–90, but in only two measures among women during this same period (Midanik and Clark, 1994). There are also signs of high-risk drinking patterns among young women, especially Whites. Mercer and Khavari (1990), in their study of drinking among college students, found significant decreases in abstention among women, significant increases in the amount of beer consumed and that women consumed more wine per occasion than men. Hughes *et al.* (1997) found that among women aged 19–25 who drink, almost 30% are heavy drinkers. Wilsnack *et al.* (1994) found 26% of women aged 21–30 reporting at least one drinking problem in the past year, compared with rates of 2–17% in older age groups.

Physically, women are more susceptible than men to the harms related to the use of alcohol. Data indicate that, with equal volumes of consumption, the risk of chronic alcohol-related diseases such as cirrhosis is greater in women than in men (Mezey *et al.*, 1988). Proposed causes include women's higher body fat, lower volumes of distribution (Dawson and Archer, 1992) and decreased ability to detoxify alcohol (Frezza *et al.*, 1990; Seitz *et al.*, 1992). A variety of medical problems such as hypertension, anemia, fatty liver, malnutrition, peptic ulcer and gastrointestinal hemorrhage have been reported to develop in alcoholic women after fewer years of drinking and less drinking per year (Ashley *et al.*, 1977), and rates of excess mortality are higher than in alcoholic men.

Women are more likely than men to receive prescriptions for psychotropic medications. They are also more likely than men to report non-prescription use of psychoactive medications such as stimulants and tranquilizers (Amodei *et al.*, 1996). The fact that women are more frequently seen in primary care settings than men offers more opportunity for diagnosis of substance abuse problems. Unfortunately, women are less likely to be asked about their substance use and only half as likely as men to have an existing alcohol problem identified by their primary care physician (Amodei *et al.*, 1996; Buchsbaum *et al.*, 1992).

Youth

Profiles of adolescents and young adults in the US reveal some important trends. Just over half of eighth graders have tried alcohol, with 80% of high school seniors and 88% of college students reporting lifetime alcohol use. Occasions of heavy drinking (five or more drinks in a row at least once in the previous two weeks) increase with increasing age, rising from 15% among eighth graders to 28% among 12th graders and 40% among college students. Alcohol use patterns in every age group have shown steady declines since 1980, with the monthly prevalence of alcohol use among high school seniors declining from 72% in 1980 to 51% in 1993. Daily use has likewise declined from 6.9% in 1979 to 2.5% in 1993, and the frequency of heavy drinking decreased by roughly one-third from 41% in 1983 to 28% in 1993. While the gender difference in heavy drinking has been diminishing very gradually over the past two decades among high school seniors, heavy drinking still remains a predominantly male phenomenon (37% vs 20%). Male college students are also much more likely than female students to report heavy drinking over the previous two weeks (52% vs 31%), with little change in these differences since 1980 (Johnston *et al.*, 1996).

Older adults

A growing body of epidemiological evidence from the past three decades indicates that the elderly are the age group at lowest risk for alcohol problems. A review of 29 studies performed between 1960–90 by Liberto *et al.* (1992) found that among older adults the percentage of abstainers is higher, the prevalence of heavy drinking and alcohol abuse is lower, and heavy drinking and alcohol-related problems, when present, are more frequent in older men than older women. Grant *et al.* (1994) found an overall percentage of DSM IV alcohol abuse and dependency of only 0.64, as compared to 3.47% among those aged 45–64 and 7.27% among those 30–44 years old. For those over 65 years of age, the prevalence of alcohol abuse or dependency is 1.2% in men and 0.3% in women (Grant *et al.*, 1994). Rates of heavy drinking are considerably higher, ranging between 11–25% (Liberto *et al.*, 1992). However, for reasons discussed below, both clinicians and researchers have raised concerns that current definitions and methods for detection of alcohol use disorders may not be adequate when applied to the elderly (Fink *et al.*, 1996; Graham, 1986; Miller *et al.*, 1991; Reid and Anderson, 1997), potentially leading to underdetection of alcohol use disorders in both clinical and epidemiological settings.

Despite more limited use of alcohol and illicit drugs, the elderly do use and at times abuse large quantities of both prescription and over-the-counter medications. Elderly patients consume a disproportionate amount of all prescription medications. Psychoactive drugs with high abuse potential (e.g. anxiolytics, sedative hypnotics and narcotic analgesics) are frequently prescribed for common geriatric conditions. The epidemiology of substance use disorders (other than alcohol) in the elderly is not well studied.

Substance abuse problems, when present, are often overlooked and under-diagnosed (Whitcup and Miller, 1987). Clinicians' index of suspicion is often low (Zimberg, 1995), and signs of substance abuse or dependency typically seen in younger patients (e.g. occupational or social disability) may be absent. An older person who is retired, does not own a car, has few family or social contacts and has few responsibilities outside the home may report few alcohol-related problems due to the change in roles related to aging (Graham, 1986). Instead, housing problems, social isolation, lack of self-care and poor nutrition may be indicators of problems associated with substance abuse. Such symptoms may be overlooked by the clinician or inaccurately attributed to effects of aging or other medical co-morbidities. Although abnormal values for laboratory tests such as mean corpuscular volume and mean corpuscular hemoglobin have been found in a majority (70%) of elderly alcoholics (Hunt *et al.*, 1988), alcohol-related illness may be less easily differentiated from the effects of other chronic illnesses and from side effects of medication. Furthermore, due to changes in body composition associated with aging (decreased lean body mass), an equivalent amount of alcohol will produce higher blood alcohol levels in older adults (Vestal *et al.*, 1977). Thus, a pattern of drinking that was non-problematic as a younger adult may become problematic as the individual ages.

While most older individuals with drinking problems begin to abuse alcohol earlier in life and experience continued alcohol-related problems in middle age and beyond, some patients develop alcoholism in later years, a syndrome often referred to as 'late-onset alcoholism' (Atkinson, 1988). Age-related losses such as retirement, loss of physical health, death and illness of friends and family, social isolation, financial problems and physical and cognitive declines that lead to barriers and inactivity may precipitate heavy drinking. While one-third to one-half of elderly alcohol abusers develop the problem at a later age (Adams and Waskel, 1991; Brennan and Moos, 1991; Liberto *et al.*, 1992), not all studies have found an association between age-related losses and the onset of alcohol use disorders (Brennan and Moos, 1991).

Drug abuse trends

Much of the population-based data on drug abuse in the US come from large government-sponsored studies or surveys similar to those used to measure alcohol use. The NHSDA collects data on trends in the use of alcohol, cigarettes, cocaine and marijuana by civilian, non-institutionalized persons aged 12 years and older. The Partnership Tracking Survey (PATS) is a series of interviews in public places whose purpose is to monitor the behavior and attitudes of young people and adults toward illegal drugs. The Monitoring the Future (MTF) surveys are annual surveys of alcohol, tobacco and other drug use conducted on a nationally representative probability sample of eighth, 10th and 12th graders in public and private schools. The NLSY, mentioned previously, collected information about both alcohol and drug use, including pregnancy and prenatal care records and follow-up physical and psychological examinations on a subsample of children born to women participants. The Youth Risk Behavior Survey (YRBS) is part of the Centers for Disease Control's (CDC) Youth Risk Behavior Surveillance System (YRBSS) which consists of national, state and local school-based surveys of ninth to 12th graders, including a national household survey. The Drug Abuse Warning Network (DAWN) monitors hospital emergency room visits and medical examiner facilities to collect information about drug-related emergency room visits and deaths. Most of the above studies identify differences in use patterns between Whites and African Americans, and some identify Hispanic users as well. As mentioned above, however, there have been no comprehensive studies of substance abuse information in Native American/Alaskan Native populations, and conclusions must be drawn from on-going school-based surveys and from regional, state and local studies.

According to data from the 1996 NHSDA, 34.8% of all respondents reported using an illicit drug in their lifetime and 6.1% in the last month. Marijuana has continued to be the most commonly used illicit drug, with 32.0% of respondents reporting use of marijuana in their lifetime and 4.7% reporting use in the past month. Cocaine (excluding crack cocaine) was the next most commonly reported illicit drug used, with 10.3% of respondents reporting use in their lifetime and 0.8% in the past month. Crack cocaine had been used by 2.2% of respondents in their lifetime, and 0.3% in the past month (USDHHS, 1998). Although cocaine use overall has declined after peaking in the early 1980s, it continues to be a significant problem, particularly among teens and young adults. The MTF studies of high school students have shown a slow but steady rise in annual and monthly use of cocaine and crack cocaine since 1990. In 1998, 5.7% of high school seniors reported using cocaine in the past year, with 2.5% reporting use of crack cocaine (USDHHS, 1998).

NHSDA data revealed lower rates of hallucinogen use, with a lifetime use prevalence of 9.7% and a past month use prevalence of 0.6%. Lifetime use of inhalants was reported by 5.6% of respondents and past month use by 0.4%. Heroin was the least commonly reported illicit drug used with a lifetime prevalence of 1.1% and past month prevalence of 0.1%. Lifetime non-medical use of stimulants, sedatives, tranquilizers and analgesics was reported by 2.7–5.5% of respondents, and past month use reported by 0.1–0.9%. Non-medical use of analgesics was the most common. Rates of past month use of any illicit drug were nearly twice as common among men (8.1%) compared to women (4.2%). The roughly 2:1 ratio persists when rates of marijuana and cocaine use are examined separately (National Institute on Drug Abuse, 1998). Hallucinogens, inhalants and prescription sedatives are more commonly abused by youths and young adults than by older adults.

African American substance use

Case study

Lakeisha W is a 25-year-old African American who presents to the Labor and Delivery suite of an urban hospital in the northeastern US in active labor with her third child. The resident on call is surprised to find that she has received no pre-natal care. However, a review of her old hospital chart from two years prior reveals that on her previous admission, she delivered a term male infant who was small for gestational age, with findings suggestive of fetal alcohol effects. Her urine drug screen was also positive for marijuana, and efforts were made to place her in inpatient substance abuse treatment. Unfortunately, the social worker was unable to find a treatment center which would accept an uninsured patient along with her two small children, and she did not keep the appointment made for her at a local outpatient treatment center two weeks after hospital discharge. Lakeisha reports that her pregnancy was unplanned, and that she 'cut way back' on her use of alcohol once she discovered she was pregnant. After denying drug use to the male resident who performed her initial evaluation, she did admit to the female medical student who followed her throughout her labor that she occasionally used crack cocaine when her boyfriend offered to share with her. Because of threats from the county Family Services Division to take her children away from her if she continued to use drugs, she did not seek pre-natal care, but now confides that she 'hopes her baby will turn out all right'. She worries because her older child is now in special education classes and is difficult to discipline, and her 18-month-old daughter is just beginning to walk and speaks only two words.

According to the 1990 census, African Americans compose 12% of the US population, or about 30 million persons (US Bureau of the Census, 1992). The African American population includes individuals from many different cultures, including backgrounds as varied as those of a Jamaican immigrant living in New York City, a second-generation Nigerian-American living in Chicago, or African Americans whose families have lived many generations in the urban ghetto of Philadelphia or a rural farm in south Georgia (Brown, 1993). Three excellent epidemiologic studies performed in the early 1980s (the previously mentioned ECA surveys (Helzer *et al.*, 1991), Herd's 1984 national survey of drinking patterns among US Blacks (Herd, 1990), and the 1984 NHHS (USDHHS, 1991)) have recently been updated by national surveys by Caetano (1997), Midanik and Clark (1994, 1995), Grant *et al.* (1994) and others to provide a comprehensive picture of alcohol problems among African Americans.

Although African Americans are more likely to abstain from alcohol use than Whites (29% vs 24% for men and 46% vs 34% for women) (Herd, 1990), total lifetime rates of alcohol abuse and/or dependency are essentially the same for both Blacks (23.7% for men, 5% for women) and Whites (23.4% for men, 4.5% for women) (Helzer *et al.*, 1991). Data from the 1992 National Longitudinal Alcohol Epidemiologic Survey (NLAES) found that the peak current (one-year) prevalence of alcohol abuse and dependency occurred at ages 18–29 (23.48%) (Grant *et al.*, 1994). This parallels current prevalence patterns in non-Blacks, whose rate of these disorders was also highest in the 18–29 age range, with rates falling gradually throughout the remainder of adult life. Several studies suggest, however, that African Americans may have greater problems than Whites in middle age. Lifetime prevalence rates from the ECA study in the 1980s suggested greater problems with alcohol abuse and dependency at ages 45–64 (32.99%) (Helzer *et al.*, 1991). Herd found that rates of frequent heavy drinking among men were highest (20%) among Black men at ages 50–59 (Herd, 1990).

The tendency toward heavy drinking during later adult years and continued heavy drinking over time may help provide some explanation for the fact that despite similar rates of alcoholism overall, African Americans suffer from significantly higher morbidity and mortality rates. As heavy drinking increases, rates of alcohol-related problems in frequent heavy drinkers increase at a more rapid rate among African American men than among White men (Herd, 1994). Consequences are also significant among African American women, whose risk of fetal alcohol syndrome appears to be six to seven times greater than among Whites (Chavez *et al.*, 1988; Sokol *et al.*, 1986). A 1998 review of death rates for alcohol-induced causes conducted by the US National Center for Health

Statistics (US Census Bureau, 1998) found that the overall mortality rate for alcohol-induced causes was 1.9 times the rate for the White population (11.5% vs 6.2%). Among the causes of these differences were higher mortality rates for cirrhosis and esophageal cancer. Despite declines in cirrhosis mortality rate in recent years, mortality rates for Blacks remain significantly higher than for Whites. Cirrhosis mortality risk for Black males is 73.8% higher than that for White males (USDHHS, 1997), and for women it is 63–77% higher (Monthly Vital Statistics Report, 1997). Incidence of squamous cell esophageal cancer, related primarily to use of alcohol and tobacco, is more than five times greater in Black men than in Whites, with Blacks showing a markedly increased carcinogenic risk from the same level of alcohol and tobacco use (Brown *et al.*, 1994). While reasons for these differences are not entirely clear, potential contributing factors include poverty, poor education, poor nutritional status and limited or delayed access to healthcare. It may also be true that continued heavy alcohol consumption in later adult life may result in greater total amounts of alcohol consumed over the lifetime, or cause continuing alcohol-related physiologic damage as drinking extends over longer periods of time. It is also possible that African Americans incur greater physiologic damage due to decreased ability to withstand or repair alcohol-related insults in older patients.

Two recent studies indicate that alcohol consumption patterns may not be decreasing among African Americans as they are in some population groups. Caetano's longitudinal study of a national multiethnic sample population found greater persistence in heavy drinking patterns among both African Americans and Hispanics than Whites over the period of 1984–92 (Caetano and Kaskutas, 1995). These findings coincide with those of Midanik and Clark, who noted that despite recent declines in the proportion of current drinkers, weekly drinkers, and heavy drinkers in the overall US population, these rates remain the same among African Americans (Midanik and Clark, 1994).

Drug use

Based on the 1996 NHSDA, 7.6% of African Americans (9.9% of males and 5.7% of females) reported using an illicit drug in the past month. Past month prevalence rates were highest for 18–25 year olds (15.7%) and lowest for those over 35 (3.8%). Marijuana use was the most common illicit drug used in the past month (6.6% of respondents), followed by cocaine (1.1%). Rates of marijuana use by African Americans were similar to Whites for those aged 25 years and younger (7.3% for 12–17 year olds, 13.9% for 18–25 year olds), but were higher than rates for Hispanic Americans and Asian Americans and approximately half the rates for Native Americans/Alaskan Natives. For African Americans over 25, rates of marijuana use were approximately 50%

higher than for Whites (9.2% for 26–34 year olds, 1.9% for those over 35) and nearly two-thirds higher than among Hispanic Americans (National Institute on Drug Abuse, 1998). Rates of cocaine and crack use for African Americans in this same age group were also twice those of White Americans, despite the fact that at younger ages (12–25), cocaine use is only half that reported by Whites (USDHHS, 1998).

Drug use during pregnancy is an important issue for African American females. According to the 1992 National Pregnancy and Health Survey (NPHS), 10.3% of African American mothers reported use of an illicit drug in the past 12 months, rates that were significantly higher than those of Whites (5.0%) and Hispanics (4.3%). Illicit drug use in pregnancy by African American mothers continues to be higher than for Whites, with 11.3% of African American mothers reporting illicit drug use during pregnancy, as compared to 4.4% of Whites. Marijuana was the most commonly reported illicit drug used (4.6% of respondents) followed by cocaine (4.5% of respondents). Crack cocaine use was far more common than other forms of cocaine use (4.1% vs 0.7%). Use of other illicit drugs was reported by less than 1% of respondents. Non-medical use of psychotherapeutics during pregnancy was reported by 3.1% of African American mothers (National Institute on Drug Abuse, 1996).

Youth

The MTF surveys found that for virtually all drugs – licit and illicit – African American high school seniors had lower rates of lifetime illicit drug use compared to Whites and Hispanics. Thirty-day and daily use rates for African American seniors were also lower than for Whites and Hispanics. The most commonly reported illicit drugs were marijuana and inhalants. Lifetime prevalence of marijuana use was 30.4% for seniors and 15.3% for eighth graders. Thirty-day use rates were 18.5% for seniors and 9.0% for eighth graders. Daily use of marijuana was reported by 3.9% of African American seniors compared to 5.5% of Whites and 4.5% of Hispanics. Lifetime prevalence rates for other drugs were less than 3% (Johnston *et al.*, 1998).

Hispanic American substance abuse

Case study
Ricardo G, a 45-year-old salesman for a distributor of photocopy machines, reports to his primary care physician for evaluation of epigastric pain. His stomach pain has been intermittent over the past year, but has increased

over the past two weeks. In the past, he got some relief from liquid ant-acid medication, but recently he has been in almost constant pain and has had to cancel two sales appointments because of pain and nausea. Upon questioning, he reveals that he often has one or two drinks at lunch or in the afternoon entertaining clients, and a 'couple of drinks' of rum or beer, or occasionally both, when he arrives home in the evening. His wife complains about his drinking, but he feels she does not understand the stress he is under at work and that having a drink with clients is an expected part of his work. Only recently has he begun to wonder whether his drinking might be a problem after his first arrest for driving under the influence of alcohol. He also admits some feelings of guilt regarding his drinking after missing his son's key soccer game because he decided to stay at the bar during Happy Hour and have 'one more drink' with his fellow sales partners.

Like the North American Black population, the Hispanic population is a diverse group representing 8% of the population, or some 20.7 million people (US Bureau of the Census, 1991). Major ethnic subgroups include Mexican Americans, who make up the largest subgroup (64%), followed by Puerto Ricans (10.5%) and Cuban Americans (4.9%). These populations are geographically concentrated in specific areas of the US with larger numbers of Mexican Americans living in the West and South-west, Puerto Ricans living in the North-east, and Cuban Americans living in Florida. In addition, some US cities have significant numbers of Hispanic Americans from countries in the Caribbean, from Central America and South America.

Important information regarding alcohol-related problems among Hispanic Americans has been obtained from numerous important studies during the past two decades. Sources of information include epidemiologic studies from the 1980s including the ECA study (Helzer *et al.*, 1991), the 1984 NHHS (USDHHS, 1991), and the Hispanic HANES (National Center for Health Statistics, 1987); regional studies by Burnam (1989), Caetano and Medina Mora (1988, 1989), Gilbert (1985, 1989; Gilbert & Cervantes, 1986); and national longitudinal studies peformed in the 1990s. These sources provide a comprehensive picture of alcohol use patterns and emerging trends in alcohol use.

Hispanic males report the highest rates of alcohol abuse and/or dependency of all ethnic subgroups studied in the five-site ECA Survey (30.02%) (Helzer *et al.*, 1991). Alcohol abuse and dependency rates are highest among males in the age group 30–44 (37.3%), with frequent heavy drinking peaking at ages 30–39 (26%). This is later than among White males but earlier than among African American males (Helzer *et al.*, 1991; USDHHS, 1991). Drinking rates vary among different Hispanic subgroups, with Mexican American men drinking more and abstaining less than either Puerto Rican or Cuban American men (National Center for Health Statistics, 1987). Several studies indicate higher rates of alcohol-related mortality among Hispanic Americans, with deaths occurring at younger ages (Gilbert, 1989). Cirrhosis deaths play a major role, with Hispanics with alcoholic liver disease demonstrating lower survival rates for reasons that are unclear (Mendenhall *et al.*, 1989). Chronic liver disease and cirrhosis are the ninth leading cause of death among Hispanics, resulting in a mortality rate of 10.0 deaths per 100 000 population (Monthly Vital Statistics Report, 1997). Death rates peak at 35.2 per 100 000, or twice the rate for non-Hispanic Whites, in the 45–64 year group.

Hispanic women, on the other hand, report some of the highest rates of alcohol abstention (45–60%) (Caetano, 1989; USDHHS, 1991) and lowest rates of alcohol abuse and/or dependency (3.85%) (Helzer *et al.*,1991) in the US population. Those who drink often do so later in life. Frequent heavy drinking peaks between the ages of 50–59 at 8% (Helzer *et al.*, 1991; USDHHS, 1991), and Hispanic women aged 45–64 are slightly more likely than White women to present with alcohol abuse or dependency (3.46% vs 2.60%). Hispanic women of Mexican American, Puerto Rican and Cuban background demonstrate no significant differences in rates of abstention or frequent heavy drinking (National Center for Health Statistics, 1987). Although Hispanic women are somewhat unlikely to develop alcoholism, those who do so show considerable vulnerability to alcohol-related medical problems. Alcoholic Hispanic women in Los Angeles report higher rates of pancreatitis than alcoholic Mexican American men, and higher rates of liver disease than either Hispanic men or Whites of either gender who are alcohol dependent (Burnam, 1989).

Education and income levels appear to exert significant influences on Hispanic American drinking patterns. Both men and women abstain less as their education increases and drink more as their income increases (National Center for Health Statistics, 1987). Patterns of migration and acculturation also appear to exert a significant effect, with recently arrived Mexican migrant men reporting rates of heavy drinking that are three to four times higher than either Mexican men (6%) or US-born Mexican Americans (9%). US-born Mexican American women, on the other hand, are only half as likely to abstain as Mexican women (33% vs 66%) (Caetano and Medina Mora, 1988). Polednak (1997) also reported significant declines in the gender difference in drinking with acculturation of Hispanic adults in Connecticut and New York, primarily due to increased alcohol consumption among women.

Drug use

According to the NHSDA, 5.3% of Hispanic Americans reported using an illicit drug in the past month, or slightly less than the US average. Marijuana was the most common illicit drug used by Hispanic Americans (3.7%). Among subgroups of Hispanics (Puerto Rican, Mexican, Cuban, Central American, South

American and other), rates of illicit drug use in the past month ranged from 7.0% for Puerto Ricans to 3.7% for 'other'. Rates of illicit drug use among men were roughly twice the rates for women (6.7% vs 3.8%). Illicit drug use was most prevalent among those aged 18–25 and lowest among those over 35 years of age. Overall rates of past month illicit drug use by Hispanic Americans were lower than all other racial/ethnic groups except Asians/Pacific Islanders (National Institute on Drug Abuse, 1998).

Women of reproductive age

Hispanic women of childbearing age (15–44) had lower rates of lifetime illicit drug use (26.2%) than either White (51.8%) or African American women (35.1%). Use of illicit drugs was generally higher for Hispanic women in non-metropolitan areas, a pattern opposite to that observed for White and African American women (National Institute on Drug Abuse, 1998). An estimated 28 100 or 4.5% of Hispanic mothers reported illicit drug use during pregnancy. Marijuana was the most common illicit drug used in pregnancy (1.5%). Rates of other illicit drug use were less than 1% (National Institute on Drug Abuse, 1996).

Youth

As high school seniors, Hispanics have the highest lifetime and annual prevalence rates for cocaine (all forms) and steroids. In the lower grades (eighth and 10th) surveyed by the MTF studies, Hispanic youths had the highest prevalence for nearly all drugs surveyed except inhalants, stimulants, hallucinogens and smokeless tobacco. Of note, these high rates are in grades prior to substantial school drop-out. Although Hispanic seniors have lower rates of drug use than Whites, these rates may be misleading since there is a higher rate of school drop-out among Hispanics (Johnston *et al.*, 1998).

Native American substance abuse

Case study
Nancy is a 15-year-old Native American girl who is brought by her mother to the reservation's health center for help with recurrent nausea, vomiting, and abdominal pain. The fourth of six children, Nancy has no significant

past medical history, other than being moderately overweight. Her symptoms first began a few months ago, but then went away after a few days without treatment. Last week her symptoms started again. Her mother decided to seek medical attention this time because the abdominal pain was a little worse and the nausea and vomiting were not going away. Her mother also wonders if she might be pregnant.

The family and social history point toward the origins of her disorder. Nancy's father was severely alcoholic and died last year in a car accident involving alcohol. Her mother does not drink but is in poor health from diabetes and worries a lot about her children. Nancy has two older sisters and an older brother. The oldest sister does not drink or use drugs, but her other sister and brother both drink and use marijuana and occasionally other drugs. Nancy had been in boarding school with her older sister, but last year moved home when a new school was built on the reservation. She had been a good student in primary school, but her grades have declined in the past two years and now her grades are average to below average.

In a private interview without her mother present, Nancy talks more openly about her substance use. One of her sisters first introduced her to alcohol at age 10, and she began using alcohol regularly at age 12. Now she goes out drinking with friends every weekend and occasionally during the week. When she and her friends go out, they drive to a store off the reservation to buy alcohol, then drive back to an isolated spot down a back road and 'party'. They usually start drinking in the car leaving the store, and when they get to their 'party' spot, they drink until all the alcohol is gone. If someone has marijuana, they all smoke it as well. Nancy always gets very drunk, and several times she has had blackouts and couldn't remember what happened at the party or how she got home. She is sexually active, and occasionally has unprotected intercourse, especially when 'partying'. She recently broke up with her boyfriend after an argument while they were both drunk. This summer, Nancy wanted to get a job, but there were few opportunities on the reservation, and she lives too far away from the nearest town where more summer jobs were available. She has thought about dropping out of school and moving in with her aunt, who lives in town, in order to get a job and help out with family finances. When asked if she has thought that her alcohol and drug use might be becoming a problem, she answers, 'Not really,' and that many of her friends drink and smoke more marijuana than she does.

Native Americans and Alaskan Natives number about 1.5 million persons, or less than 1% of the population of the US, with the greatest concentrations living on reservations and in pueblos in the South-west. Cultural diversity among Native Americans is profound. There are more than 500 separate tribal entities within the US and Canada, speaking more than 200 distinct languages

(Group for the Advancement of Psychiatry, 1996; Mail and Johnson, 1993), and there are few genetic, linguistic or cultural features that would distinguish them as a single entity for epidemiologic purposes. Most Alaskan Natives live in isolated villages and towns, where 52% of Native Americans living in the 48 contiguous states live in urban areas. Many 'urban' Native Americans are transient, moving back and forth from tribal village or reservation, depending on job, family, education, health and recreational circumstances (Group for the Advancement of Psychiatry, 1996).

The history of alcohol problems in native North American populations is unique because, prior to the arrival of Europeans, distillation was virtually unknown. North of the 35th Northern latitude in Mexico, fermented beverages were found only among two South-western tribes: the Tohono O'Odham, who made sacred wine, and the Apachean peoples, who made a secular cactus beer (Bourke, 1894: Opler, 1941). Some authorities suggest that White colonists provided models of drinking as an expression of power and prestige for Native Americans to emulate, while others note that alcohol was readily absorbed into cultures where notions of power were associated with altered states of consciousness (Group for the Advancement of Psychiatry, 1996).

While there are no comprehensive epidemiologic studies of substance abuse among Native Americans, numerous studies of specific tribes and individual communities, as well as admission data from formal alcohol treatment programs, indicate that abuse of alcohol and other substances is a major problem.

Alcohol use patterns

It is important to emphasize that in some tribal groups, there is little alcohol use or abuse, although this is generally the exception rather than the rule. At times there are stark differences between neighboring populations. For example, most Hopis of the South-western US do not drink, viewing drinking as irresponsible and a threat to cosmic harmony (Levy and Kunitz, 1974), while among neighboring Navahos, 55% drink and 14% are heavy drinkers (Group for the Advancement of Psychiatry, 1996). Alcohol use generally begins during the teenage years (Leung *et al.*, 1993), and while there are many abstainers and many heavy drinkers, there are relatively few moderate drinkers (Lemert, 1982; May, 1982). Many Native Americans engage in abrupt and intense bouts of episodic or binge drinking, during which large quantities of alcohol are consumed almost non-stop over a period of several days (Robin *et al.*, 1998; Westermeyer and Baker, 1986). Episodes often end only after money runs out (Westermeyer, 1979) or unconsciousness prevails (Curley, 1967; Rozynko and Ferguson, 1978). While some anthropologic and ethnographic analyses have depicted binge drinking as a recreational, normative, traditional and often positive behavior, more detailed quantitative studies have found high correlations between binge drinking and multiple social, work, physical and legal problems, as well as violence, alcohol dependency, and other psychiatric disorders (Alvarado and Seale, 1997; Robin *et al.*, 1998; Westermeyer, 1976). Factors which appear to increase the harm related to alcohol use include the fact that drinking is the primary recreational activity in many Native American communities, as well as the belief that alcohol abuse is the acceptable way of drinking and that problems arising from drunkenness may be excused or taken for granted 'because the person was drunk' (Heath, 1989; Moss, 1979). In the 1980s, several investigators described alcoholism rates several times higher than in the general population, with the majority of patients with alcohol problems demonstrating alcohol dependency (May, 1982; Silk-Walker *et al.*, 1988; Westermeyer, 1982). Three recent studies have corroborated these findings, documenting alcohol abuse and dependency rates of 75–83% among men and 39–51% among women (Leung *et al.*, 1993; Manson *et al.*, 1992; Robin *et al.*, 1998). Several studies indicate that urban Native Americans drink more heavily than those who remain in rural areas (Beltrame and McQueen, 1979; Weibel-Orlando *et al.*, 1984). Other studies have described spontaneous remission in significant numbers of patients after 15–20 years of drinking, with some researchers reporting remission rates as high as 50–60% (Burns *et al.*, 1974; Leung *et al.*, 1993; Medicine, 1982).

Consequences of heavy drinking

Numerous observers, clinicians and investigators would agree with Andre's assessment of alcohol abuse as 'the most widespread, severe and all-encompassing health and social problem among American Indians today ...' (Andre, 1979). In some areas, Native Americans are dramatically over-represented in the alcohol and drug treatment population. In Alaska, for example, Alaskan Natives make up 65% of the treatment populations, but only 17% of the general population (Weibel-Orlando, 1985). Five of the top 10 causes of death among Native American adults (accidents, cirrhosis, alcoholism, suicide, and homicide) are strongly related to alcohol abuse and dependency, accounting for more than one-third of all adult deaths (Institute of Medicine, 1990). In part due to increased cirrhosis mortality rates, mortality from alcoholism among Native Americans is three to four times the US national average, with deaths occurring at earlier ages (USDHHS, 1990). One positive trend is the fact that since 1969 the overall rate of death due to alcoholism has been steadily decreasing (Mail and Johnson, 1993). Alcohol-related mortality is strikingly high among Native American women, whose death rate actually exceeds that of males in the 15–24 age group (Indian Health Service, 1990). Cirrhosis mortality is more than triple the rate among Black women and six times the rate among White women (Johnson, 1978).

Women of childbearing age

Fetal alcohol syndrome (FAS) and fetal alcohol effects are also more frequent than among the general population (USDHHS, 1990), with FAS rates documented at three to four per 1000 births, or 30 times the rate among Whites (Chavez *et al.*, 1988; Egeland *et al.*, 1998). Women who abuse alcohol frequently give birth to more than one alcohol-damaged baby (May *et al.*, 1983).

Drug use

Based on NHSDA data, Native Americans and Alaskan Natives report the highest past month illicit drug use rate (11.3%) of all of the racial/ethnic groups studied. As with other racial/ethnic groups, rates for men (15.1%) were roughly twice rates for women (8.0%). Age-related patterns of use parallel the other racial/ethnic groups with highest rates in the 18–25 age range (25.4%), and falling off sharply for those over 35 years of age (3.7%). Marijuana is the most common illicit drug used overall (10.0%), with approximately one out of four Native Americans/Alaskan Natives between 18–25 reporting marijuana use in the past month (National Institute on Drug Abuse, 1998).

Adolescent substance abuse

Problems of substance abuse among adolescents are highlighted in the case study described above. Alcohol problems among adolescents are extremely prevalent (Lamarine, 1988; Oetting and Beauvais, 1989), with some studies indicating higher rates of alcohol-related problems among both males and females when contrasted with Whites (May, 1982). Alcohol is often combined with other drugs, particularly inhalants and marijuana, and use is often earlier and more frequent than among White adolescents (Mason *et al.*, 1985). Available data indicate that marijuana is the most frequent drug of abuse, with as many as 88% of adolescents in some areas reporting a history of marijuana use. Inhalant abuse may start by fourth grade or earlier, with use continuing through the end of high school in as many as one-third of adolescents surveyed (May, 1982).

Substance abuse in primary care

The high rates of substance abuse across all ethnic boundaries and the high morbidity of this disorder demand the attention of primary care providers. Those who provide primary care are in a unique position to identify and help patients with drug and alcohol problems, who are twice as likely as the general population to consult a primary care physician (Rush, 1989). Despite the fact that up to 20% of visits to primary care physicians are related to substance abuse and/or dependency (Bradley, 1994), primary care detection rates average only 45–65% of those affected (Buchsbaum *et al.*, 1992; Bush *et al.*, 1987; Moore and Malitz, 1986). Those patients detected are usually those in the most advanced stages of the disease, where significant sequelae remain, even if substance abuse recovery is achieved. The urgency to improve primary care detection has led to efforts not only to identify patients affected by substance abuse and dependency, but also to identify disease-free patients whose high-risk patterns of drug and alcohol use place them at risk of developing substance abuse problems.

Patterns of high-risk alcohol consumption

Key research findings have led to a clearer definition of two alcohol use patterns which are linked to alcohol-related problems: higher levels of daily alcohol use (more than two to three drinks per day) and intermittent binge drinking (the consumption of five or six drinks during a single drinking episode, where a standard drink is defined as one 12-ounce [360 ml] bottle of beer or wine cooler, one five-ounce [150 ml] glass of wine, or 1.5 ounces [45 ml] of distilled spirits). Investigators have found a clear dose response curve above two to three standard drinks per day for the risk of cirrhosis, alcohol-related cancers, heart disease, strokes, trauma, and depression (Anderson *et al.*, 1993). Midanik *et al.* (1996) found that 20% of North American men and women who drink an average of three drinks per day met ICD-10 criteria for alcohol dependency, and Room and colleagues (1995) found that 25% of Canadians drinking 2.5 drinks per day had experienced two or more adverse consequences of drinking. As noted above, women appear to be more sensitive to alcohol-related consequences than men and less able to detoxify alcohol.

The risk of binge drinking, even on an intermittent basis, has also been clearly documented. Three separate studies have demonstrated that persons who consume more than five or six drinks per day, even on an intermittent basis, are at increased risk of experiencing alcohol-related problems (Casswell *et al.*, 1993; Dawson and Archer, 1993; Room *et al.*, 1995; Single, 1994). Binge drinking also increases the risk of certain acute medical problems such as cardiotoxicity and cerebral infarction (Ashley *et al.*, 1997).

Because of the clear correlation between these drinking behaviors and alcohol-related problems, current typologies for classifying patient drinking behavior now include the category of at-risk drinking (*see* Figure 1.1). Patients 'at risk' for problems with alcohol outnumber alcohol-dependent patients four to one (Institute of Medicine, 1990). Although they drink less and have fewer problems than alcohol-dependent persons, because of their greater numbers, healthcare costs are considerably higher for this group. Sometimes referred to as 'alcohol/drug misusers', they are less severely affected than alcohol-dependent patients, usually drinking and/or using other drugs less frequently and in smaller amounts. Physical consequences from their misuse are usually minimal. Such patients are generally employed, socially stable, and able to meet their major daily responsibilities (Kahan, 1996). Often, these individuals have more insight regarding the relationship between their substance use and its adverse consequences and demonstrate less denial in the clinical setting. Guidelines currently in use define high-risk drinkers as those who:

- exceed safe drinking limits (two to three drinks per day for men and one to two drinks per day for women)
- drink in high-risk situations such as pregnancy, while driving a motor vehicle or while taking medication which interacts with alcohol
- engage in binge drinking.

Two studies performed in primary care settings in the US (Fleming *et al.*, 1998) and New Zealand (McMenamin, 1994) found that 9–10% of patients fell within the at-risk category, and that these patients could be identified using simple screening methods. This population appears to be highly amenable to risk reduction intervention. As noted in the above definitions, there are slight differences from country to country on the levels of daily or weekly alcohol consumption which are considered 'at-risk' (*see* Table 1.1). While guidelines proposed by the British Medical Association (British Medical Association, 1995) and the

Table 1.1   Recommended safe drinking limits (weekly consumption)

	Men	*Women and older adults*
Canadian Centre on Substance Abuse and NIAAA (US)	<14 drinks	<7 drinks
British Medical Association and World Health Organization	<21 drinks	<14 drinks

References: ARF/CCSA, 1994; BMA, 1995; NIAAA, 1995; Saunders *et al.*, 1993a.

World Health Organization (Saunders *et al.*, 1993a) for defining at-risk drinking are slightly higher than those in use in Canada (Addiction Research Foundation/Canadian Centre on Substance Abuse, 1994) and the US (National Institute on Alcohol Abuse and Alcoholism, 1995), we believe that the evidence for increased alcohol-related harm for individuals who observe the higher limits is compelling (Midanik, 1996; Room *et al.*, 1995), and that the lower limits are more appropriate for identifying high-risk drinkers in the primary care setting. Methods for using the guidelines in health promotion and risk reduction will be further discussed in Chapter 6.

Conclusion

Substance abuse is a widespread disease that affects a major percentage of the population worldwide. Although alcohol remains the most widely abused substance, the abuse of other psychoactive substances continues to proliferate, and in many areas the concomitant abuse of alcohol and other drugs now represents the norm. The burden of this disease stretches across boundaries of geography, age, gender and ethnicity to touch individuals from almost every conceivable kind of background. While the cost of this disease in terms of dollars is staggering, the financial cost may indeed be outweighed by the human suffering of patients and those whose lives they touch. Research findings of the past two decades have provided us with clearer and clearer definitions of how substance abuse disorders affect differing population groups, and have also identified at-risk substance use behaviors which put patients at increased risk of developing such disorders. This is extremely valuable information for the patient-centered clinician, who can utilize this information to provide health promotion to low-risk patients, prevention with patients who demonstrate at-risk alcohol and drug consumption, and treatment where problems of abuse and dependency are already present.

2

Alcoholism: pathophysiology of a disease

Jack R Woodside Jr

Editor's introduction

The first component of the patient-centered method distinguishes disease and illness. Effective care requires clinicians' understanding and facility with both concepts. Dr Woodside explores the 'body-as-machine' portion of the first component as he leads readers toward an appreciation of the illness experience. Exploring evidence and implications of the disease concept of alcoholism, this chapter begins with a review of the historical evolution of the concept of alcoholism as a disease: speeches by Abraham Lincoln and editorials from the JAMA in the 1890s, writings from the founders of Alcoholics Anonymous (AA), and the American Medical Association's (AMA) declaration of alcoholism as a disease in the 1950s. This is followed by a review of the scientific evidence supporting the disease concept. Investigations demonstrating genetic transmission including twin and adoption studies are presented along with research leading toward biochemical markers, and 'valid' biological bases for disease. Dr Woodside also reviews emergent literature describing the neurobiologic role of the mesolimbic dopamine system in craving and in the maintenance of drinking behavior. Case studies demonstrating patterns of inheritance facilitate his discussion, particularly as this relates to the perspective of an alcohol-dependent person attempting to recover. The disease concept is described as playing a valuable role in mitigating shame and promoting acceptance of a recovery process. Taking this broader perspective, the disease concept has important implications for society's approach to alcoholism, the responsibility of the healthcare industry, and third-party payers.

This chapter uses the terms 'addiction' and 'substance dependency' as synonyms, describing the diseased state without specifying the mood-altering substance (or substances) involved. The term 'alcoholism' is used when citing specific writings where the authors referred to alcohol dependency only. In this chapter, the term 'alcoholism' (or 'alcohol dependency') refers to a manifestation of addiction where dependence on alcohol is most prominent. Alcoholism and dependence on other mood-altering substances are considered specific subsets of the broader, inclusive disease of addiction. This concept will be expanded on later in this chapter.

It is often assumed that the approach to alcoholism as a disease is a relatively modern concept. Frequently, the AMA's declaration of alcoholism as a disease in 1956 is cited as a landmark event (American Medical Association, 1956). However, the concept of alcoholism as a disease has fallen in and out of favor periodically in the past. For example, in his 1842 speech to the Temperance Union, Abraham Lincoln referred to alcoholism in terms very similar to those used by modern proponents of the disease concept. Stating, 'The victims to it [intoxicating liquor] were pitied, and compassionated, just as are now the heirs of consumptions, and other hereditary diseases' (Lincoln, 1842). He presaged modern neurobiology's characterization of alcoholism as a disorder of appetite in the following sentence: 'For the man to suddenly, or in any other way, to break off from the use of drams, who has indulged in them for a long course of years, and until his appetite for them has become ten or a hundred fold stronger, and more craving, than any natural appetite can be, requires a most powerful moral effort'. Lincoln was describing a view of alcoholism as a hereditary disease expressing itself as a disordered, abnormally strong appetite.

This disease concept was widespread during the last half of the 19th century resulting in the formation of institutes and asylums for the treatment of alcoholism. Dr Leslie E. Keeley announced in 1879, 'Drunkenness is a disease and I can cure it'. Over 120 Keeley Institutes were opened in North America and Europe (White, 2000). The American Association for the Cure of Inebriety (AACI) was founded in 1870 and the *Journal of Inebriety* appeared in 1876 (White, 2000).

In 1894 there appeared in the *Journal of the American Medical Association* an article entitled 'The Disease of Inebriety'. In this article, the author specifically refers to the dichotomy of viewing alcoholism as 'Moral Delinquency' as opposed to disease. Interestingly, the author assumed that if alcoholism were a disease, it would be more likely to be curable than if it were a moral delinquency. Again, with an uncanny resemblance to modern neurobiology, the author likened alcoholism to a disordered appetite, not unlike hunger or thirst, which would result in 'urgency for relief so great that the will has not the power to resist'. This author, like Lincoln, speculated that the appearance of a failure of the will could instead be the result of a uniquely strong appetite.

In the first half of the 20th century opinion moved away from the disease concept towards a view of alcoholism and addiction as moral issues. This was coincident with the passage of the Harrison Narcotic Act in 1914 and prohibition (ratification of the 18th amendment to the Constitution) in 1919. It wasn't until the last half of the 20th century that the disease concept and medical treatment of the addictions became widespread again.

A consensus panel reached a definition of alcoholism, which was published in the *Journal of the American Medical Association* in 1992 (Morse and Flavin,

1992). This definition described alcoholism as a 'primary, chronic disease with genetic, psychosocial, and environmental factors influencing its development and manifestations'. This definition was important not only in asserting that alcoholism is a disease with biologic components but emphasizing alcoholism as a primary disease, not simply the consequence of other underlying problems; for example, depression or social stress.

One characteristic of a disease is a clearly recognizable set of signs and symptoms (Lewis, 1994). One commonly recognized description of addiction can be found in the fourth edition of the *Diagnostic and Statistical Manual* (DSM IV). DSM IV describes substance dependency as a pattern of behavior without specifically addressing the underlying cause of the behavior. According to the DSM IV there are seven criteria for substance dependency, any three of which are sufficient to make the diagnosis. The first two criteria relate directly to biologic tolerance and withdrawal, which are more likely to be features of dependence on opiate or sedative hypnotic drugs. Other classes of substances produce little or no tolerance and withdrawal. The remaining five criteria, however, describe behavior resulting from loss of control of substance use. One example is use despite significant impact on the individual's life and health. These criteria reflect the external behaviors that are associated with the internal phenomena of craving. The unifying feature of the modern disease concept of addiction is this disordered craving for the use of the substance (or substances), which results in the external behaviors that we recognize as addiction. The DSM IV does not distinguish between alcoholism and dependence on other substances. In fact, the criteria for substance dependency are the same for all of the drugs of dependence. This is congruent with modern thinking, which looks at addiction as a disease independent of the specific substance (or substances) involved. An increasing number of patients treated for addictions are dependent on multiple substances. In other patients the disease will evolve over time, substituting one substance for another. One example is the alcoholic who quits drinking by substituting benzodiazepines. One challenge for addiction medicine is to explain how a variety of chemicals with a wide range of pharmacologic effects can all produce the same pattern of behavior we term addiction. In the 1980s the American Society for Alcoholism and Other Drug Dependence (AMSODD) changed its name to the American Society of Addiction Medicine (ASAM) to reflect this common nature of dependence on alcohol and other drugs.

A disease also has a recognizable natural history, with some variation from one individual to another. One frequently discussed issue is whether this disease persists for a lifetime, so that despite remissions, the individual carries a lifetime vulnerability to relapse. A second, related question concerns the feasibility of a patient with addiction returning to moderate use of mood-altering substances (e.g. controlled drinking). George Vaillant, a Harvard psychiatrist, has arguably the most comprehensive data on the natural history of alcoholism. Vaillant

(1996) analyzed data collected over a 50-year span (from adolescence to retirement age) about two groups of White males in Boston. The 'core city sample' was 456 men from inner-city Boston. The 'college sample' was 268 Harvard University sophomores, followed until 70 years of age. Vaillant observed that alcohol use fluctuated over a lifetime and was not inevitably progressive. Although many alcohol abusers returned to controlled drinking, this was not a stable state and most eventually relapsed to heavy drinking or achieved stable abstinence. However, after five years of abstinence, return to drinking was rare. Of interest is that although the 'core city' group began drinking at an earlier age, and was more likely to become alcohol dependent, it was twice as likely as the college sample to achieve stable abstinence.

Another characteristic of a disease is that it has a biological basis (American Medical Association Committee on Alcoholism, 1956). The biological evidence for the disease of addiction comes from several fronts, including genetic studies, animal models for alcoholism, biological markers for the disease and direct neurobiological studies of the brain's motivation and reward systems. The familial nature of alcoholism has been recognized since ancient times, as evidenced by the quote from Plutarch, 'drunkards begat drunkards' (Goodwin, 1985). However, the familial nature of the disease does not necessarily prove a biogenetic basis since environmental influence is also transmitted from parents to children. A particularly vivid example is the fact that regional accents are transmitted from parents to children. However, it is unlikely that a genetic *locus* for southern twang will be found. In order to separate genetic from environmental influences, two different approaches are taken: twin studies and adoption studies. Twin studies are based on the observation that identical twins share 100% of their genetic material whereas fraternal twins share 50% of their genetic material (similar to any other first-degree relative). Therefore, if a disease were 100% genetic-based (and has complete penetrance, such as hemophilia), in the case of identical twins if the disease affected one twin, the other would be affected 100% of the time. In the language of twin studies, this would represent 100% concordance within the twin group. The concordance between fraternal twins for a purely genetic disease would be much lower (similar to that for other first-degree relatives). In 1960, Kaij conducted twin studies and discovered that among identical twins there was 74% concordance for alcoholism, whereas fraternal twins demonstrated only 32% concordance (Kaij, 1960). Clearly, the fact that identical twins show double the level of concordance reflects a strong inherited genetic component for alcoholism. However, the concordance was somewhat less than 100%, which also reflects the fact that factors other than genetics are operative. These findings were essentially confirmed in a study in 1981 by Hrubec who found a concordance among fraternal twins of 13%, which was also doubled for identical twins with a concordance of 26% (Hrubec and Omenn, 1991). Underlying twin studies is the assumption that because twins are born into a household at the same time, they are exposed to identical environmental influences during their upbringing. One criticism of twin studies is that the environment experienced by the twins may be more similar for identical twins than it is for fraternal twins. For example, both parents and acquaintances will be more likely to treat identical twins in a similar fashion than they would treat fraternal twins. Identical twins are more likely to be dressed alike or even mistaken for one another because of their similar appearance, personality and temperament. Therefore, it is possible that the increased concordance observed for identical twins could be a result of their environments being more similar than is found with fraternal twins. In 1987, Kaprio examined the influence of this bias and concluded that although it is a concern in the case of alcoholism studies, genetics still account for 36–40% of the transmission of this disease (Kaprio *et al.*, 1987).

Another line of investigation looks at adoption records. These studies take advantage of the fact that the genetic influence of the biologic parent is divorced from the environmental influences of the adoptive parents. In particular, study of the biologic offspring of an alcoholic parent, when raised in an adoptive home without alcoholism, should allow the dissection of the influences of genetics and environment. The best known of these studies has derived from investigations conducted in Scandinavian countries. In these countries, adoption records are available to investigators so that biologic parents can be readily identified. In addition, centralization of health records in these countries allows access to information about the presence of alcoholism in the adoptee and the biologic parent, as well as the adoptive parents. In 1973, Goodwin examined records in Copenhagen, Denmark, covering adoptions between 1924 and 1947 (Goodwin *et al.*, 1973). He identified 55 adoptees who had a parent who had been hospitalized for alcoholism. In this group, 18% of the adoptees later developed alcoholism themselves. This is in comparison to 78 adoptees who served as a control who had no evidence of alcoholism in their biologic parent. The second control group expressed a 5% incidence of alcoholism. Therefore, Goodwin demonstrated three times the incidence of alcoholism among adoptees who had a biologic parent who suffered from alcoholism, even though this parent had little or no environmental influence on the upbringing of the child. In addition, Goodwin looked at the presence of other psychiatric diagnoses and was unable to find an association with the presence of alcoholism. Specifically, there was no association between alcoholism and depression, neuroses or other personality disorders. Cloninger conducted a similar experimental design with adoption records in Stockholm, Sweden, between 1930 and 49 (Cloninger *et al.*, 1981). Cloninger's group was larger, including 862 adoptees of which 151 were alcoholics. Cloninger's findings effectively confirm Goodwin's results that the incidence of alcoholism was increased threefold when there was a biologic parent suffering from alcoholism. In addition, the large size of Cloninger's group allowed an interesting subgroup to be identified. Cloninger identified 31 cases where the offspring of a biologic parent with alcoholism was adopted into a home where alcoholism was also present. This group then experienced the combined genetic and environmental influence of alcoholism. Rather than showing an additive effect, this subgroup actually showed a decrease in the incidence of alcoholism from 18% to 13%. Because of the small group size, this reduction failed to achieve statistical significance. However, the data suggest that the presence of alcoholism in a child's environment might actually be protective towards the development of alcoholism in later life. Harburg provides independent evidence that children's exposure to a problem drinking father results in children that are more likely to abstain or be light drinkers (Harburg *et al.*, 1990). This is certainly consistent with anecdotal observations of children of alcoholics, where it is not uncommon to find individuals so negatively influenced by the damage caused by alcoholism in their family that they consciously decide never to drink. They therefore never expose themselves to the possibility of alcoholism, even though they may have inherited the genetic susceptibility. Critics of adoption studies point out that the biologic parents have some environmental impact during the first few months of life, and the pre-natal environment carries the potential to influence the offspring. Also, adoption agencies' placement of children is not an entirely random process and could conceivably introduce subtle and obscure bias. However, despite these concerns, adoption studies do seem to provide strong evidence that a biologic transmission of alcoholism takes place.

These early studies by Goodwin and Cloninger examined primarily men and provide little evidence of genetic transmission of alcoholism in women. Some researchers concluded that alcoholism in women was not genetically transmitted. Alternatively, the social and cultural influences on the expression of alcoholism in women may have left women alcoholics less visible in the early studies. In 1992, Kendler provided strong evidence that genetics play a major role in alcoholism in women (Kendler *et al.*, 1992). In a study of 1030 twin pairs there was an increased concordance for fraternal twins as compared to the population. This effect was markedly stronger for identical twins, suggesting a strong genetic influence. Kendler also observed that identical twins do not have 100% concordance for alcoholism even though they share identical genetic material. This implies that factors other than genetic, such as environmental and social influences, play a role. Based on their data, Kendler *et al.* (1992) estimated that between 50–61% of the liability for alcoholism is inherited.

If indeed alcoholism is genetic, then in theory it should be possible to breed selectively to produce alcoholic (or non-alcoholic) offspring. Although selective breeding studies in humans are not ethical or feasible, rats can be selectively bred for alcoholism. In 1979, Li demonstrated what appeared to be purebred strains for alcoholic rats (Li *et al.*, 1979). Li took standard Sprague Dawley laboratory rats and offered them a choice of water and dilute alcohol solution. He observed those rats that seemed to prefer the alcohol solution as well as those rats that seemed to avoid it. These two groups of rats were then separated and selectively inbred until, after several generations of inbreeding, he produced pure strains of alcohol-preferring (P) and alcohol non-preferring (NP) rats. These rats seemed to be stable down through subsequent generations of breeding and in many ways resembled human behavior of alcoholism. In particular, the rats would prefer the alcohol solution even if it were administered directly to the stomach by a gastric tube (Waller *et al.*, 1984). This demonstrated that the rats were selecting the alcohol solution for its effect rather than simply a taste preference. The alcohol-preferring rats also given free access to alcohol would drink until they developed tolerance and dependency similar to human alcoholics. Perhaps most interesting, the alcohol-preferring rats were shown to have reduced serotonin and dopamine levels in their brains (Murphy *et al.*, 1982, 1987). These reductions and neurotransmitter levels were observed in alcohol-preferring rats before they had ever been exposed to alcohol. So, Li had been able to demonstrate not only a genetic trait in rats that in many ways resembles human alcoholism but was also able to associate this trait with abnormalities in brain neurochemistry.

A second line of evidence derives from the supposition that if alcoholism is an inheritable genetic trait then there must be a biologic abnormality among alcoholics that is the physical reflection of the alternate genetic material. This leads to the search for biologic markers for the disease of alcoholism. Part of the difficulty with identifying biologic markers is separating the influence of years of alcohol exposure itself from characteristics that are inborn and pre-date alcohol use.

Henri Begleiter approached this dilemma by examining young sons of alcoholics who had not yet themselves been exposed to alcohol. This group of sons of alcoholics (labeled FHP for 'family history positive') is at increased risk from alcoholism (Begleiter *et al.*, 1984). The genetic studies cited above suggest that the first-generation offspring should have an incidence of alcoholism of approximately 30% compared to the 8–10% incidence in the general population. If the biologic markers were present in a greater percentage of individuals in this FHP group as compared to the control ('family history negative') group (FHN), then the conclusion was that the biologic marker was the result of an inherited difference rather than simply the toxic effects of alcohol. Specifically, Dr Begleiter examined event-related potentials, a specialized form of an electroencephalogram (EEG). Event-related potentials record the EEG for a short period of time following a sensory stimulus. This sensory stimulus can be visual in the form of a flash of light, or auditory in the form of a click delivered through headphones or even a somatosensory stimulus delivered to an extremity. These sensory stimuli are repeated many times and the resulting EEGs are electronically added together. With multiple repetitions, the random neuronal activity taking place in the brain will tend to cancel out in the summation, and a waveform emerges that reflects the specific neuronal response to the sensory stimulus. Begleiter looked at the neuronal response to both visual and auditory stimuli that resulted when the stimulus changed in character; for example, when a vertical line flashed on a screen suddenly changed to a horizontal line or when an auditory tone changed pitch. Begleiter observed that this waveform was significantly different in the case of alcoholics. The magnitude of the EEG wave 300 msec following the stimulus was significantly reduced in amplitude in alcoholic individuals. More significantly, Begleiter observed that in the young sons of alcoholics this reduction in the P 300 wave was also present, which implies that this reduction is a trait marker for alcoholism rather than simply the toxic effects of alcohol itself.

Another interesting line of investigation looks at enzyme activity in the cells of alcoholics. Tabakoff examined the enzyme adenylate cyclase in platelets of alcoholics and controls (Tabakoff *et al.*, 1988). Baseline activity of adenylate cyclase was the same in alcoholics and controls. However, alcoholics showed less stimulation of the enzyme's activity by guanine and fluoride. This trait remains present in alcoholics despite sustained abstinence, which implies that the trait is independent of the direct effects of alcohol. Even more intriguing is the observation that the magnitude of this difference continues to increase over the years in abstinent alcoholics, completely apart from exposure to alcoholism. There is considerable anecdotal observation that alcoholism seems to be a progressive disease throughout the lifetime of the individual. Many feel that this progression continues to take place even in alcoholics who are abstinent so that if a relapse occurs after many years of abstinence, the disease reappears in an increasingly severe form. The evidence of this enzyme abnormality progressing even during periods of abstinence would lend some biologic credence to this concept of disease progression.

The biologic markers described above may be linked genetically, but not related, to the etiology of alcoholism. The question then remains, 'what exactly is inherited?'. Shuckit and Gold observed that sons of alcoholics (a high-risk group for alcoholism) were less sensitive to the effects of alcohol as measured by subjective effects and body sway in response to a dose of alcohol (Shuckit and Gold, 1988). They hypothesize that this attenuated reaction to alcohol may result in a reduced tendency to regulate alcohol intake and lead to heavy use. In a follow-up study 10 years later, Shuckit (1999) found that more of the sons of alcoholic fathers had developed alcoholism (34% vs 13%). What's more, the sons with the strongest attenuation of response to alcohol were the most likely to have developed alcoholism during the follow-up interval. In a study of EEG response to alcohol, Volavka found that subjects whose EEGs had the smallest response to a dose of alcohol were the most likely to have developed alcoholism 10 years later (Volavka *et al.*, 1996). Many alcoholics report that from the beginning of their drinking careers they were able to drink large quantities of alcohol with relatively little effect (Shuckit, 1999). A similar decrease in response to alcohol was observed in mice (Crabbe *et al.*, 1996). These mice had a mutated gene that prevented production of one of the subtypes of the serotonin receptor ($5HT_{1B}$). These mice were less sensitive to the effects of alcohol and also were observed to drink double the amount of alcohol. Crabbe concluded (like Shuckit) that the reduced sensitivity to the effects of alcohol resulted in a loss of regulation on the amount of alcohol intake. Recent work by Shuckit has looked at associations of neurotransmitter genotypes with level of response to alcohol in his original study group (Schuckit *et al.*, 1999). Interestingly, both a serotonin transporter gene and a GABA receptor gene were associated with low response to alcohol and increased risk from alcoholism in his group of subjects.

If indeed the disease of addiction is the result of a genetic defect that is manifested in the biology of the individual, then the natural question is where this defect in biology resides. Since the underlying defect in addiction appears to be an inordinate craving for the mood-altering substance, then it is natural to look at those regions of the brain that are the source of normal appetites. In particular, attention has turned to the mesolimbic dopamine system of the brain, which includes the ventral tegmental area, the nucleus accumbens and the pre-frontal cortex. This system is often described as the motivation or reward system in the brain and mediates biologic appetites such as hunger, thirst and sexual drive. These appetites lie at the basis of survival for the individual and the species and are correspondingly located at a rudimentary level in the brain. They are operating in neuronal systems well below the cerebral cortex and conscious thought. Corresponding to their relationship to basic survival, they produce appetites (such as hunger and thirst) which are powerful, and in their more severe forms ultimately irresistible. The neurons of this mesolimbic dopamine system, with cell bodies in the ventral tegmental area and synapses in the nucleus accumbens, are primarily dopaminergic. It is becoming clear that many, and probably all, substances of abuse influence this mesolimbic dopamine system at one site or another. For example, GABA receptors are located on the axons of these dopaminergic neurons. GABA receptors are believed to be the site of action of benzodiazepines as well as a likely site of action for alcohol. Opiate receptors are located on the terminal axons of interneurons synapsing with these dopaminergic neurons, as well as on postsynaptic membranes and the dopaminergic synapses in the nucleus accumbens. Cocaine, on the other hand, appears to block the re-uptake of dopamine and the synapses of nucleus accumbens, allowing augmentation of dopamine's effect on the post-synaptic neuron. This augmentation of dopamine levels by cocaine is probably the most direct and obvious example of a drug of abuse enhancing the activity of this reward or pleasure system. Receptors for tetrahydrocannabinol (THC) have recently been identified and presumably will be found to influence this system at some level.

The disease hypothesis is that those individuals who have inherited the genetic susceptibility to substance dependency have a mesolimbic dopamine system which is uniquely susceptible to the influences of mood-altering drugs.

It is clear from receptor studies that sustained drug use produces profound perturbations in these neuronal systems. For example, dopamine receptor density is known to be decreased by sustained use of cocaine. This would be consistent with a prolonged enhancement of dopamine's effect in the synapse, which could lead both to a reduction in numbers of dopamine receptors as well as a down-regulation of the sensitivity of these receptors to the effects of dopamine. Positron emission tomography (PET) scans of cocaine addicts reveal significant decreases in dopamine receptor numbers. It is interesting to note that the decreases in receptor density are observable even after four months of abstinence from cocaine use (Volkow *et al.*, 1993). This implies that the alteration in brain function that results from cocaine use persists after many months of abstinence. This helps explain the presence of significant craving and risk of relapse even after several months of abstinence from drug use. These persistent changes in receptors could also help explain protracted withdrawal (Satel *et al.*, 1993). Protracted withdrawal is based on the clinical observation that subtle signs of withdrawal can be observed after six to 12 months of abstinence. These receptor findings illustrate why the effects of drug use persist for far longer than it takes the body to physically eliminate the substance from the body.

The existence of the mesolimbic dopamine system also provides a unifying concept that explains another intriguing clinical observation regarding substance dependency. It is that relapse rates over time for widely diverse substances such as alcohol, nicotine and heroin are quite similar (Jorenby, 1997). Abstinence rates overall are difficult to interpret since they are influenced significantly by the selection of the underlying population, the type of treatment for substance dependency that was administered, aggressiveness of follow-up and whether or not pharmacological screening is used to confirm abstinence. However, long-term abstinence rates from alcohol, smoking and narcotic use seem to fall within the 20–30% range and are remarkably similar for these three diverse substances. Also, a plot of incidence of relapse *vs* time expressed in months produces relapse curves that again are remarkably similar for these three substances. The similarities in relapse among these very different substances of abuse suggest strongly that there is a single disease that is underlying all three patterns of dependency. Also, mice strains that show high ethanol preference also are susceptible to other drugs of abuse such as nicotine and opiates (George, 1987). Further evidence comes from drug-priming experiments in animals. Drug priming is the observation that a drug dose can reinstate drug-taking behavior in animals after a lapse in drug taking (Gerber and Stretch, 1975). Priming doses can be given by direct injections into the brain and are most effective when injected into the ventral tegmental area and nucleus accumbens of the mesolimbic dopamine pathways (Stewart and Vezina, 1988). Furthermore, 'cross-priming' occurs where, for example, priming doses of amphetamine reinstate opiate self-administration. The recognition of the mesolimbic dopamine system then provides a neurochemical mechanism for addiction that can produce a single pattern of dependency for diverse substances of abuse (Gardner, 1997).

This understanding of the mesolimbic dopamine system offers a biologic correlate for the unitary concept of addictions. In particular, substance dependency seems to have remarkably similar manifestations independent of the actual substance being abused. For example, the DSM IV criteria for substance dependency are the same, regardless if the drug of choice is alcohol, cocaine, sedative drugs, hallucinogens or stimulants. More and more drug treatment professionals recognize that it is unusual to find an individual who is abusing a single substance. What is more common is for individuals to be using multiple substances and to frequently substitute the use of one substance for another based on availability and other factors. Until recently, it was difficult to understand why the five classes of drug abuse (sedative hypnotics, opiates, stimulants, hallucinogens, and inhalants) which have quite diverse pharmacological effects all seem to result in a very similar pattern of substance dependency. The neurobiology would suggest all of these substances are altering the mesolimbic dopamine system in a way that results in the generation of a disordered appetite associated with the use of the drug. This appetite, in susceptible individuals, can reach sufficient strength to manifest itself as addiction. Addiction is a craving for the drug that eclipses the ability of reason and will to modify it. These individuals are experiencing a craving which is similar in all respects to the hunger of a starving individual or the thirst of an individual trapped in the desert. When viewed from this perspective, an individual's use of substances could assume a degree of importance in their life that could result in their sacrificing health, job, family and indeed all valued aspects of their life.

One criticism of the biologic disease concept of addiction is that if we are dealing with a disease, then why is it that traditional methods of treatment have been essentially behavioral or even spiritual (as in the case of AA)? A biologic disease would seem to require a biologic treatment. Recently, there have been several advances in the pharmacological treatment of alcoholism, some of which seem to influence this basic biochemical mechanism for craving. Probably the earliest example of pharmacological treatments is the use of disulfiram (Antabuse). Disulfiram blocks the biochemical pathways for metabolism of alcohol, such that when an individual consumes alcohol the toxic metabolite formaldehyde accumulates in their body. The formaldehyde in turn produces flushing, nausea, vomiting and an overall distressful state that is intended to act as a deterrent to drinking. Although disulfiram has been around for some time, it has had little dramatic effect on the treatment of alcoholism. A large Veterans Administration Study (VAS) observed that patients with alcoholism taking disulfiram had relapse rates that were essentially unchanged (Fuller *et. al.*, 1986). They did observe, however, that those individuals who did relapse tended to drink less if they were receiving disulfiram. Another objection to the use of disulfiram is that the reaction that occurs with alcohol use can be a severe cardiovascular stress, so that it is contraindicated in those people who have significant heart disease. In any case, disulfiram appears to offer at best aversive therapy for drinking rather than addressing the underlying neurochemical mechanisms that result in craving.

More promising has been the observation that naltrexone (Revia), an opiate receptor blocker, has a beneficial effect on relapse rates in alcoholics. Naltrexone was originally proposed for the treatment of opiate addiction, since the administration of this orally active blocker renders an opiate addict unable to obtain pharmacological effect from the use of heroin. It was originally felt that if an individual was unable to achieve any pharmacologic effect from administering heroin, in time the behavior would extinguish. Results in the real world were not universally successful, in part because the success of the treatment was dependent upon the individual's adherence to taking the naltrexone. Investigation of naltrexone's effect on alcoholism has been promising. Volpicelli studied naltrexone as an adjunct to treatment for alcohol. At 12 weeks following treatment, 23% of a group receiving naltrexone had relapsed as compared to 54% of a group who received a placebo (Volpicelli *et al.*, 1992). This and another study specifically observed that those who tried alcohol while taking naltrexone drank less, resulting in fewer drinking days and less total amount drunk (O'Malley *et al.*, 1992). Therefore, those patients who 'slipped' and took a drink were less likely to progress to a full relapse. In a later study, Volpicelli demonstrated that this was the result of naltrexone's blocking the subjective pleasurable effects of alcohol (Volpicelli *et al.*, 1995). It also appears that naltrexone reduces craving for alcohol. Recent results with nalmefene (another opiate antagonist) demonstrate similar effects in alcohol dependency (Mason *et al.*, 1999). This confirms that the effects are the result of opiate receptor blockade rather than an idiosyncratic effect of naltrexone. At first appearance it is difficult to understand how an agent that blocks opiate receptors could have an effect on individuals suffering from alcohol dependency. Opiates and alcohol are two very different compounds, the first operating at the level of endorphin receptors in the brain and the second operating at the level of biologic membranes and probably GABA receptors. However, both endorphin receptors and GABA receptors impact the mesolimbic dopamine reward system. Animal research demonstrates that opiate receptor blockers reduce alcohol-stimulated dopamine release in the nucleus accumbens (Benjamin *et al.*, 1993). It appears that naltrexone is altering alcohol's effect on the basic neurobiology of reward.

A new drug under study and currently available in Europe, calcium bisacetylhomotaurinante (acamprosate), is also effective in treating alcohol dependence. This compound binds the GABA receptors, so its effects on alcohol dependency are perhaps easier to appreciate. A large (272 patients) German trial of acamprosate demonstrated, at 48 weeks following treatment, 43% of the individuals receiving acamprosate were abstinent which was significantly higher than the 21% abstinence rate in the placebo group. Both naltrexone and acamprosate seem to be compounds whose site of action is the mesolimbic dopamine system and impact the underlying mechanisms of craving responsible for alcoholism.

Apart from the possibility of the pharmacological treatments for addiction, this unitary disease concept offers significant implications both for health professionals treating this disease and individuals who are suffering from the effects of the disease. In particular, the moral view of addiction as a personal weakness contributes to the significant stigma that surrounds addiction. The shame and guilt associated with addiction is a significant barrier to the treatment of individuals suffering from this disease. Stigma also serves as a justification for healthcare professionals dismissing what is clearly a difficult and often frustrating condition to address. The stigma associated with addiction is not unique, however. Many psychiatric illnesses suffer from a similar stigma. Those individuals who view depression as a personal failing will be less likely to seek help for and even admit the symptoms of this treatable condition. Likewise, individuals suffering from addiction who believe it to be a moral failing will be less likely to admit the problem or ask for help. Therefore, the concept of the disease of addiction serves to reduce the barrier of stigma.

The book *Drug-Impaired Professionals* by Coombs contains the following quote from a nurse:

> 'The disease concept is the most powerful thing. When I got fired the first time the head nurse told me 'you are a terrible person, and I never want to see you again.' But when a compassionate person told me in a caring way that I was a sick person who needed help, not a bad person, I went into treatment. I went home and started calling hospitals' (Coombs, 1997).

For this person, casting her addiction in the model of disease carried an implied promise of treatment that would not have been possible for immoral behavior. Many object that the disease model of addiction relieves the individual from responsibility for their behavior. Coombs points out that the disease model implies that the individual is responsible for seeking treatment and maintaining on-going treatment to sustain remission. A pharmacist quoted in the book states, 'You aren't responsible for your disease, but you are responsible for your recovery' (Coombs, 1997).

3

'Sinking in a gentle pool of wine': substance abuse and literature

Sonya H Cashdan and James M Turnbull

Editor's introduction

Advancing from the disciplines of literature and psychiatry, Doctors Cashdan and Turnbull combine efforts to offer readers a perspective into the world of mood-altering substance use as portrayed in literature and the arts. Opening with a review of classical Greek and Roman writings, Talmudic and Christian theology, Nordic mythology and New World spiritual beliefs, these authors culminate with an examination of contemporary literature and media.

The intent of this chapter is to explore mood-altering substances in Western cultures as depicted in literature and films. This chapter explores the illness experience when drugs have been used to alter mood, to self-medicate, to rebel or to enhance pleasure, while providing readers with literature designed to enhance appreciation for the role of gender issues in recovery. Biographical and autobiographical materials are submitted as resources and as a means of exploring the illness perspectives of people suffering from substance abuse and addiction. Reviewing print, music and film media, these authors offer novel insights into how abusers perceive themselves and their worlds and how the inhabitants of their worlds view them, thereby showing us how literature and film can assist us to understand the experiences of people addicted to alcohol and its impact on their families and friends.

Since substance abuse of any sort incorporates a web of motivations, circumstances, difficulties, reactions and emotions, the reservoir of qualitative and subjective experiences expressed in non-medical literature offers valuable insights to healthcare providers. Whether 'serious' or merely entertaining, the multifaceted literature of popular culture can vividly convey the subjective elements of substance abuse, addiction, denial and the illness experience itself.

Evidence of humanity's ambivalent relationship with mind-altering substances, as well as the terrible tenacity of addiction to those substances, percolates through the arts and literatures of popular culture, from mythology to the present millennium. In fact, modern writers from every literary genre often claim drugs and/or alcohol as their Muses in general, much as 'classical' Greek and Roman creators claimed by name the appropriate Muse for enhancing a particular talent.

Substance abuse in early literature

Literature and the arts reveal that different societies evinced widely differing beliefs about mental, emotional or sensory alteration. *The Odyssey* (Homer, 1963), for example, includes among the various trials endured by the homeward-bound Odysseus an episode in the land of the Lotus Eaters. Consuming lotus flowers first caused delightful dreams and luxurious lassitude; addiction to the opium-like flowers, however, produced reactions of pleasant lethargy so deep that partakers often died because eating mere food took too much energy. Greeks who could not get their 'fixes' died slowly if not forcibly removed from their fields of dreaming; Odysseus lost several sailors to the lure of the lotus. Similarly, the dark and silent waters of the river Lethe, across which the dead must pass to reach Hades and from which they must drink to forget their former lives, caused such a profound forgetfulness that even if miraculously rescued from death, the drinkers experienced perpetual amnesia. Unlike the lotus and the waters of Lethe, however, alcohol could be boon rather than bane (Bulfinch, 1998).

Graeco-Roman culture, with its pantheon of Bacchic and/or Dionysian deities and religious rituals, incorporated alcoholic beverages into worship, celebration and sacrifice. The more intoxicated the worshippers or celebrants, the deeper their supposed communion with their gods. Wine fueled the religious frenzies of the Bacchantes, priestesses who insured the next year's abundant harvest by chasing an equally intoxicated Year-king into the hills, coupling with him as long as his stamina allowed, and then tearing him apart so that his blood (and the wine which they poured out to the gods) would enrich the soil (Bulfinch, 1998).

In the dual-class Graeco-Roman society (masters and slaves, even in the temples), masters drank whenever they wished, tended by slaves who indulged only when permitted, under penalty of scourging or death for disobedience. With the passing centuries, consumption of alcohol for pleasure rather than for worship slid into outright abuse and spread even among the legendary Roman legions, eroding the discipline and prowess they had attained.

Comments in the *New Testament* (*Matthew* 24:48–49; *Luke* 7:23, King James Version), while Rome still ruled much of the known world, prove that Christians certainly considered drunkenness a major problem among all the pagan peoples of the time, with several Greek, Roman and Asian cities condemned by name. Lead poisoning, assert historians, contributed to the fall of the Roman

Empire: the raw, strong wines imbibed so frequently leached lead from serving and storage vessels. Even the dissolution of empires could not pierce the haze of alcohol addiction or break its bonds (Gibbon, 1932).

Substance abuse and religion

Norse mythology displayed a similar focus upon alcohol as celebration, symbol, or reward; the central structure of a Viking village was its mead-hall. Boasting promises of conquest and various heroic deeds, made publicly and formalized with numerous shouted toasts and upended drinking horns, sealed a warrior's word before his leader and his peers. Libations consumed and/or poured onto altars for the Norse pantheon accompanied prayers for victory; similar toasts and sacrifices sanctified the funeral celebrations for leaders and heroes. Warriors who died in battle anticipated swift passage to the eternal Mead-hall of Valhalla, riding behind statuesque Valkyries who brandished spears as they galloped skyward on flying horses. Vikings who died on raiding expeditions expected to join their heroic brethren, perpetually downing foaming, never-empty beakers of mystical mead in the haven of heroes. Eternal rewards meant eternal roistering with noble companions and with equally boisterous Norse deities, all of them served by toothsome, mead-bearing shield maids. Like Norse deities, Egyptian deities such as Isis and Osiris, the mated goddess and god of life and death, received offerings of wine, beer and hallucinogenic plants. Priests and priestesses of the various gods and demigods burned hemp with incense on altars and in censers; they also consumed wine mulled with sense-altering plant essences in order to move quickly into vision-seeking trances. In the great embalming temples, priests and priestesses supervised the addition of mood-altering substances to the vats of natron and spices used for mummification and conservation (Bulfinch, 1998).

Old Testament writings further confirm the secular records of humanity's love/hate relationship with alcohol (*Leviticus* 10:8–10; *Numbers* 6:3–4). The book of *Proverbs* (23:31–32) enjoins wise folk not to 'look upon the wine when it is red [undiluted]' and enumerates the curses of excessive drinking, including complete loss of appropriate composure, public shame and cosmic-class hangovers. In particular, the 23rd chapter of *Proverbs* details the subjective experience of drunkenness: bruises, red eyes, staggering, hallucinations, confusion and such nausea that the abuser feels caught in the rigging of a storm-tossed and very small boat.

On the other hand, the *Pentateuch* (Jewish scriptures also called the *Torah*, the first five books of the *Old Testament*) contains catalogs of instructions for believers and still more for the Levitical priests, explaining the appropriate uses of wine in worship, healing, cleansing and sacrifice. Harvest and 'first fruit' offerings required a tithe of wine along with the sacrifices of grains, oil, spices and fattened herd-beasts. In addition to precious metals and costly accoutrements, the measure of a man's wealth always included his vineyards, his wine presses and his stored jars of wine.

In a similar vein, the *New Testament* bewails pagan alcohol abuse, chastising Christians who over-indulge (I *Thessalonians* 5:6–8; I *Timothy* 3:2–3; *Luke* 1:15), yet the first recorded miracle of Jesus details how he transmuted water into wine at a poor man's wedding feast in Cana of Galilee (*John* 2:1–11) . One song from the *New Testament*-based musical and film *Jesus Christ Superstar* (Jewison, Universal, California) contains the wistful wish of the worried disciples that 'all [our] trials and tribulations' would sink temporarily 'in a gentle pool of wine'. Even the rather formal and solemn St. Paul, who roundly condemned almost any activity that smacked of frivolity, urged his disciple Timothy to 'take a little wine' as medicine for his stomach problems. Similarly, the Good Samaritan 'poured on oil and wine' to cleanse the wounds of the man who had been robbed, beaten, and left for dead. In his teachings, although Jesus firmly chastised drunkards, He referred frequently to spiritual epiphany as 'a taste of new wine' (*Matthew* 9:15). And, in a ritual now central to Christian liturgy and worship, Jesus used wine at the Last Supper to symbolize the blood which he would willingly shed for the eternal 'health' of his followers.

In the West, oral literatures as well as the recorded tribal histories of Native Americans (North, South, and Central) abound with references to mind-altering substances, almost always in a religious or spiritual context. The Toltecs, Incas, Mayas and Aztecs, for example, used wine even in blood-sacrifice rituals, as part of an offering to the gods and occasionally as an anodyne for the pains of the human sacrifices. For centuries prior to the European introduction of powerful fermented beverages, Native Americans had used herbal stimulants and intoxicants of various sorts, sometimes for healing and sometimes in worship or celebration. Shamans regularly incorporated hallucinogens in 'vision quests' and meditation, often in tandem with fasting, steam baths, and/or other physical stresses. Although Carlos Castaneda later admitted that 'some' of his series of books about the Yagui shaman Don Juan Matus contained more fiction than fact, the books nevertheless garnered considerable interest in the 1960s and 1970s. In particular, *Teachings of Don Juan* (Castaneda, 1974), *Separate Reality: further conversations with Don Juan* (Castaneda, 1972), and *Power of Silence: further lessons of Don Juan* (Castaneda, 1987) extolled the virtues of peyote as a mind-altering substance, useful for opening an aspirant's consciousness to communion with the infinite. Thousands of seekers, most more concerned with sensation than with spirituality, 'popped' peyote buttons.

Drunkenness/intoxication as part of, or as a result of, important spiritual and healing rituals carried few if any social stigmas for Native Americans. Ingestion of intoxicants opened the minds of seers, prophets and postulants to messages from the gods, eased the pain of the wounded, the ill or the dying and allowed even non-shamans an occasional glimpse of the divine. However, as European settlers enslaved, robbed and displaced Native Americans, forcing them onto reservations and shredding their traditions, alcohol use for those ethnic groups mutated into deadly and pervasive alcoholism. At first called 'medicine-water' because its early effects mimicked those of other hallucinogens, alcohol earned the name 'fire-water' because of its destructive and addictive properties.

Substance abuse in modern literature

In the 20th century, the term 'literature' has broadened to mean considerably more than printed books and magazines. Now we have flyers, documentaries, commercials and 'infomercials,' song lyrics, films and television series, e-mail and television 'magazines,' plays, sermons, billboards, bumper stickers, musicals, speeches, newspapers, 'fanzines,' in-house newsletters, books on tape, story-telling festivals, interactive adventure games for computers, etc. Today's audiences read, listen to, view and often create their own literature. The literature of popular culture further chronicles and illustrates not only society's ambivalent relationship with mood-altering substances, but also the subjective experience of being 'under the influence'.

'Substance abuse', even as a denotative diagnostic term, carries pejorative as well as medicosocial connotations. Classified as a disease, one addiction among many which plague modern society, alcoholism permeates every level of that society, presenting a continuing challenge to healthcare providers. To further complicate treatment, women who abuse alcohol have largely been 'closeted' until the last quarter of the 20th century; tens of thousands have endured for decades as 'functional alcoholics' whose lives have masked their addictions. Getting patients to recognize and admit that substance abuse problems actually exist becomes difficult indeed when abusers live safely behind societal walls. The medicinal toddies and brandies of 19th century America have given way to the aperitifs and cocktails of the 20th century, as alcohol retains its veneer of social acceptability and even of glamour. Early film icons (the original screen sirens of the 'talkies') invariably appeared on-screen either with martini glass (and long, slender cigarette holder) in hand or knocking back a shot with the guys.

In addition to such walls of respectability or glamour for women, popular culture abounds with conflicting messages about substance use/abuse in general. During Prohibition, for example, a whole sub-culture based upon asserting one's individual freedom by flouting that particular amendment flourished, with the US government as the villains. The anonymous folk song *Away with Rum*', for example, highlighted the absurdities of various anti-alcohol crusades by citing 'a man in the gutter with crumbs on his face' (from the yeast in cookies), a man 'eating fruitcake and then getting tight' (from rum flavoring), and the reeling recipient of a back-rub: 'just think of the liquor your body soaks in!' Tales of moonshine, 'bathtub gin', 'revenuers' as 'bad guys' and moonshiners as heroes, speakeasies, and bootlegging live on, mostly in films such as '*Thunder Road*' and in music.

The lyrics of popular music have frequently portrayed drinking as a part of courtship, a sort of adjunct to romance, with many a flattering alcohol-based metaphor for the female object of affection. 'Easy listening' songs of the 1930s and 1940s, for example, often depicted alcohol in a rosy glow: according to the singing lover, a desirable woman, like an excellent martini, possessed a definite 'slam bang tang' which he fully appreciated. Another lovely woman spins in another singer's thoughts 'like the bubbles in a glass of champagne'; she 'intoxicates' his soul like some 'sparkling burgundy brew' or 'the kicker' in a mint julep. One song urged lovers to celebrate 'the moonlight cocktail', adding kisses and a star to the alcoholic contents as desired.

Anonymous college drinking songs such as '*Wine, Wine, Wine*' (a song which lends itself to quickly improvised verses in between rowdy roarings of the chorus), '*It's Rum, Rum, Rum,*' and '*Drunk Last Night; Drunk the Night Before*' treated alcohol abuse as a highly amusing collegiate rite of passage and a sure way to rev up school spirit before the big game. Many a college drinking game, either with alcohol as reward or with shots of liquor as penalties, still encourages copious consumption as part of the college experience. Anonymous folk songs, many of them originating in the British Isles and 'Americanized' through the years, reveal still more contradictory ideas about drinking. '*Three Jolly Coachmen*' praised 'the man who drinks dark ale and goes to bed quite mellow' while warning that the abstemious man who drank only 'water pure' would 'die before October' (Kingston Trio, Capital Records, California). In 18th and 19th century England, before the advent of reliably pure water and antibiotics, 'water pure' was a relative term, and mildly alcoholic beverages were often safer than water, but not in 20th century America, when the song gained popularity. Similarly, the whaling song '*Early in the Morning*' offers a series of unpleasant consequences in answer to the Captain's question, 'What shall we do with the drunken sailor?' The sailors who shout for colorful punishments are, of course, drunk themselves, but they can still function, which their cohort cannot. Later folk songs extolled the virtues of *Mountain Dew* and *White Lightnin'*, advising entrepreneurs to 'get you a copper kettle [and] a copper coil' so they could lie beneath a juniper tree in the moonlight while they watched their fortune distilling into whiskey jugs. During Prohibition, illegal and unlicensed manufacturing of liquor could earn someone a quick fortune, but not in mid-20th century America, when those songs became popular. Beginning in the early 1960s, such songs as The Kingston Trio's gentle *Scotch and Soda*, in which the bemused lover feels 'higher than a kite can fly' (Kingston Trio, Capital Records, California); Judy Collins's lively *Bottle of Wine*, with the audience singing along on the 'when ya gonna let me get sober?' chorus (Collins, Electra Records, New York); and Roger Miller's rowdy *Chug-a-lug*, after which action the 'chugger' wants 'to holler hi-dee-ho!' despite his burning 'tummy' (Miller, Hal Leonard Publishing Corp., Milwaukee), had moved from the hoot-nanny, the university, and the Big Bands to the recording studio, the television studio and the airways.

The Prohibition idea of government as enemy grew more pervasive in the 1960s, with such New Age gurus as Dr Timothy Leary and the poet Alan Ginzberg popularizing the notion that LSD, even more than alcohol, allowed users to see 'the truth' about life and government. Leary urged truth-seekers to 'turn on, tune in, and drop out' of 'The Establishment', a message also promoted by acid-rock music and by the cult rock musical *Hair* (Forman, United Artists, California), which director Milos Forman transformed into the just-as-cultish 1979 film of the same name. Protest, acid- and folk-rock songs urged listeners to join 'the mellow life' by smoking marijuana and experimenting with other mood-altering substances. An earlier musical (without the 'in your face' attitude of *Hair*), *Porgy and Bess*, featured the silkily sinister pusher Sportin' Life, smoothly portrayed by Sammy Davis Jr. in Otto Preminger's 1959 film version (Preminger, Samuel Goldwyn Co., California). Sportin' Life plied his trade by promising that '*It Ain't Necessarily So*'. Conventional morality could cease to burden those who used his 'happy dust'.

Mixed messages continued. In numerous pseudoshamanistic and pseudo-autobiographical book-length manifestos, as mentioned earlier, New Age wanna-be-guru Carlos Castaneda (1972, 1974, 1987) lauded the efficacy of hallucinogens as tools for comprehending the mysteries of life. The 1969 film *Easy Rider*, directed and co-written by Dennis Hopper (Hopper, Columbia Pictures Corp, California), pictured dope-users merely as harmless pilgrims in search of meaning for their lives, motorcycle-mounted wanderers plagued by the narrow-minded moralists of 'The Establishment'. Hippies touted 'flower power' while ingesting opium poppy derivatives; their inhibitions decimated by drugs and alcohol, they proclaimed 'free love' and sexual revolution while generating the now-deadly and still growing epidemic of STDs which plagues 21st century life.

Some films focused on substance abuse in Hollywood, often becoming merely film versions of tabloids rather than honest examination of a problem. Director Mark Robson's melodramatic 1967 film *Valley of the Dolls* accurately portrayed the hedonism of Hollywood women addicted to alcohol and 'dolls', various prescription drugs, the uppers and downers which fogged the aching clarity of their empty up-and-down lives. The film offered no moralizing or condemnation, but neither did it offer any solutions or replacements for drug abuse and alcoholism. Another bleak portrait of life in Hollywood, *A Star Is Born* (its 1937 original (Selznick International Pictures, California) and later remakes), documented the downfall of a brilliant but alcoholic actor, ending in his suicide. Neither the original nor the remakes suggest alternative ways of combating stress. The audience leaves saddened but entranced by alcoholism as artistic fate rather than as disease. Although director Mike Nichols's 1966 film treatment of Edward Albee's *Who's Afraid of Virginia Woolf?* (Nichols, Warner Brothers, California) focused on non-Hollywood characters, it brought into vivid and searing relief the emptiness and desolation of lives enslaved by alcohol, via the superb acting talents of Elizabeth Taylor and Richard Burton, themselves alcoholics. As Burton's character forces Taylor's character to confront the truth (they have no son except in drunken fantasies) the film offers a final valid insight: only in confronting fact and accepting reality can the alcoholic begin to heal.

Other popular films, based firmly in biography, chronicled the drug-and-alcohol-doomed lives and accidental or deliberate deaths of rock stars. *The Rose* (Rydell, 20th Century Fox, California), with its blurry camera sweeps, low-angled shots, and strobe-like lighting, as well as its creative use of Dolby sound systems, conveyed both the dissolution and despair of its Janis Joplin-based protagonist and the altered auditory and visual perceptions caused by substance abuse, particularly by hallucinogenics. Similarly, director Oliver Stone's *The Doors* (Stone, Imagine Entertainment, California) chronicles the rise and fall of Doors' lead singer and song-writer Jim Morrison, vividly sung and acted by Val Kilmer. The film draws viewers painfully close to Morrison's drug-and-alcohol saturated final days, blurring on-screen images and fuzzing sounds to illustrate alcohol-induced hallucinations and alcohol-ravaged senses. In a wry twist, famed choreographer Bob Fosse wrote and directed his autobiographical treatment of substance abuse in the entertainment world: he prophesied his own death from drugs and alcohol in the award-winning musical and movie *All That Jazz* (Fosse, 20th Century Fox, California). Converting his life into art, Fosse actually distanced himself from his addictions; he also added to the drug/ alcohol/creativity myths.

In the last decade of the 20th century, several films have depicted the ultimate alienation of the abuser, even an abuser who at first sought a sense of community in drugs or alcohol. *Leaving Las Vegas* (Figges, MGM, California), for example, features a woman who, in an act of genuine compassion, lets her traumatized lover deliberately and definitively drink himself to death. So entrapped by his disease is he that the power of his addiction persuades his non-addicted lover to accede to his death-wish. His passivity about life transmutes into a passion for death, a passion laced throughout with self-loathing exacerbated by the alcohol which slowly kills him.

The film *Face/Off*, despite its unlikely exchange of identities, does convey the frenetic pace and irrational 'reasoning' of a drug-hyped assassin, as well as the rapidly shifting perceptions and bumbling reflexes of his drug-addled undercover double (Woo, Paramount, California). Dark clothing, banks of mirrors, reflective windows, echoing acoustics, flickering lights, sprays of shattering glass and blurred and shifting camera work all imitate the subjective experience of the substance-shocked protagonists.

In a different milieu, the huge and precedent-setting music festival at Woodstock in 1969 featured scores of groups and individual singers who praised the consciousness-raising powers of drugs and alcohol, especially of 'natural' substances such as peyote buttons and the ubiquitous, 'harmless' herb marijuana. Both before and after Woodstock, a new crop of songs continued the drug-praising trend: *White Rabbit*, heavy with Alice-in-Wonderland allusions and imagery, enjoined listeners to 'feed your head' in order to stay calm and in control; the anonymous *Talking Vietnam Potluck Blues* touted marijuana as the bridge between opposing armies, the solution to the Vietnam conflict. Some songs added the festival itself to their paeans: Joni Mitchell, for example, in a song named for the festival, sang of attending Woodstock 'to try and get my soul free' because 'we've got to get ourselves back to the Garden [of Eden]' (Mitchell, Warner Brothers Records, New York). Bouncy melodies carried lyrics urging listeners to grab a 'reefer' and go 'one toke over the line', to take a 'magic carpet ride' courtesy of hallucinogens, to accompany the singers to 'strawberry fields' of drug-induced sensation, to join them on their *Yellow Submarine* (named for a popular submarine-shaped capsule), or to try the 'crystal blue persuasion' of LSD.

Another genre, Country & Western music, seldom praises drugs and rarely mentions increased levels of 'understanding', but it does focus consistently on the necessity of alcohol consumption for enduring the proverbial broken heart. Willie Nelson pleads, 'Whiskey River, take my mind', begging alcohol to have mercy on the singer and dull the pain of love gone wrong (Nelson, Columbia Records, NC). Another singer pleads for *Red, Red Wine* to ease his loneliness. *There Stands the Glass* commends the magic elixir that will soothe the singer's fears, dry his tears, ease his pain, settle his brain and dim his troubles and it's only his first glass on that particular day (Pierce, Time-Life Music, Richmond, VA). Tex Ritter professes his devotion to *Rye Whiskey*, even though that 'villain' has been his downfall: 'Kick me and stomp me, but I love you fer all' (Ritter, Capital Records, California).

Other songs, sung by women, praise various liquors by name: Johnny Walker, Jack Daniels, Jose Cuervo, and Jim Beam are men who not only liven up an evening but also never desert their women, as various absent lovers have done. One bereft singer of the 1960s begged, 'Brandy, leave me alone', Brandy being both the man-stealing woman and the singer's new anodyne. In a similar mood, one singer mourns, 'Whiskey, if you were a woman, I'd kill you for taking my man'; Loretta Lynn expresses the opposite sentiment to her alcoholic mate: 'Don't come home a-drinkin' with lovin' on your mind!' (Lynn, Time-Life Music, Richmond, VA).

If Country & Western songs do not praise the efficacy of alcohol as a desperation refuge or an emotional anesthetic, they often extol its supremacy as a means of celebration. In *The Big Book of Country Music*, Richard Carlin comments on country music's swing from 'Americana' to alcohol: 'songs about mother, home, and church were hardly acceptable to an audience drenched in beer and lusting after loose women . . . ' (Carlin, Penguin, New York). One songs proclaims 'Cigareets [sic], Whiskey, and Wild, Wild Women' as a boozy trinity to which the singer avidly clings, despite his admission that 'They'll drive you crazy; they'll drive you insane' (http//www.roughstock. com/cowpie/songs, n.d.) [Unless otherwise cited, quotes from Country & Western songs are taken from that Internet address.] Merle Haggard's *Okie From Muskogee* eschews drug use but proudly proclaims that 'White Lightnin's still the biggest thrill of all' (Haggard, Time-Life Music, Richmond, VA). Hank Williams, Jr mopes musically because none of his formerly rowdy friends want to 'get drunk and get loud'; to his disgust, they've all settled down.

Moving from life to death, one lorn lover predicts, in title and chorus, that *If Drinkin' Don't Kill Me, Her Memory Will*; he has drunk so much to forget her that he could use 'the blood from my body' to 'start my own still'. In a lighter vein, *Prop Me Up Against the Jukebox When I Die* requests that another singer's friends place a cold beer in his dead hands for his after-life enjoyment, since he's not yet ready to leave his tavern for Heaven. On that same topic, the Gatlin Brothers song *There is no Beer in Heaven* asserts that, such being the case, the singers prefer an alternative after-life destination.

Alcohol and detective novels

As mentioned above, the Western world's ambivalent attitude toward substance use/abuse permeates the writings of authors who claim alcohol or other mind-altering substances as their Muses. Edgar Allan Poe, founding father of both the American mystery story and the American detective novel, manifested in his own life the dualism of society's attitudes toward substance abuse. Most of his fiction and poetry paints a bleak landscape of despair, the details as murky as drug- or alcohol-induced perceptions. An alcoholic for certain, an opium addict probably, Poe died penniless in Baltimore at 40, leaving a reputation for extreme politeness when sober but cynical, sarcastic rudeness when drunk (Goodwin, 1990).

This twin personality, which displays the dark side of the artist, typifies many writers. In *Alcohol and the Writer* (1990), Professor Donald Goodwin notes that Robert Louis Stevenson describes such a duality, as Dr Jekyll agonizes about his dissolution in the novel *Dr Jekyll and Mr Hyde*:

> whereas in the beginning the difficulty had been to throw off the body of Jekyll, it had been of late gradually but decidedly transferred to the other

side. I was slowly losing control of my original and better self and becoming slowly incorporated with my second and worse self.

The 'split', of course, resulted directly from Jekyll's experiments with a mind-altering substance, which he had invented and ingested.

Sir Arthur Conan Doyle, the physician who created Sherlock Holmes, described a deductive genius quietly addicted to cocaine. In the film *The Seven Percent Solution* (Ross, Universal, California), Alan Alda as Sherlock Holmes receives treatment for this addiction from none other than Dr Sigmund Freud. In several stories, the narrator Dr Watson observes that Holmes finishes his case, finds himself in need of mental stimulation lest he succumb to boredom, and reaches upward with his long arms and 'slender fingers' for the cocaine bottle residing on his mantel. Watson records the habit, but does not indulge. Nor does he pass judgment (Goodwin, 1990).

Perhaps the many authors who followed in the footsteps of Doyle made their detectives lovers of alcohol because Holmes was a drug addict, or because those who hunt criminals need 'painkillers' or even because they themselves had/ have a love of 'getting high'. In *Alcohol and the Writer*, Professor Goodwin, who has spent his professional life studying and writing about alcohol and its abuse, analyzes eight authors whom he suspects or knows to be alcoholics. One such writer, Georges Simenon, created the French detective Inspector Maigret of the Sûreté. Maigret spends much of his time both on-duty (interviewing suspects, having lunch with his staff) and off-duty with his friend the doctor, drinking. Writing of his experience in the US, author Simenon asserts that:

> ... the crowds cease to be anonymous, the bars cease to be ordinary ill-lit places, the taxi drivers complaining or menacing people. It is the same for all the big American cities: Los Angeles, San Francisco, Boston .... From one end of the country to the other there exists a freemasonry of alcoholics. (Goodwin, 1990)

Despite America's apparent freewheeling views of alcoholism, however, Simenon claims that although he drank for 20 years in France without feeling any remorse, he became ashamed of his drinking for the first time after moving to the US. Simenon stopped drinking altogether in his 50s, without losing his Muse, and showed no signs of alcoholism in his 80s.

Derek Raymond, one unabashedly alcoholic writer of mystery novels who died just a few years ago, invented an unnamed anti-hero detective who featured in such novels as *Dead Man Upright* and *I Was Dora Suarez*. Although that unnamed detective did not exhibit definite alcoholism, Raymond once confessed to a writer at *The Sunday Telegraph* that he wrote all his novels in a local pub, where he stayed continuously drinking from the time they opened until they closed (Goodwin, 1990).

Several authors of mystery novels have depicted their detectives as recovering alcoholics. JP Beaumont, the policeman in JA Lance's series, is a recovering alcoholic; so is Dave Robicheaux, the Sheriff's deputy in the stories by James Lee Burke (who won an Edgar for one novel in the series). Perhaps the best-known recovering alcoholic character in the mystery genre is detective Matt Scudder, who frequently attends AA meetings as well as being a sponsor for other recovering alcoholics. Scudder's creator, Lawrence Block, reveals little personal information on the flyleaves of his novels, but his fiction exhibits his in-depth knowledge of AA's methods and philosophies; it also reveals his intimate familiarity with the fantasies and temptations of the alcoholic (Goodwin, 1990).

Alcohol as muse

Although Ernest ('Papa') Hemingway often featured hard-driving drinkers in his novels, and although he was widely known to appreciate alcohol in quantity, he never attributed his creativity to his consumption. Two writers, however, stand out as having made it clear that they would not have been as well remembered or have written so well had they not been alcoholic: William Faulkner and Charles Bukowski. Goodwin writes of Faulkner: 'Most people are probably unaware that William Clark Faulkner wrote most of his novels at night while his faithful servant whisked away the flies and supplied him with the bourbon which he consumed in large amounts' (1990). Faulkner started to manifest symptoms of alcoholism, including delirium tremens and hematemesis, in his early 30s. Although hardly a day passed from his adolescence to his death when he was not intoxicated, he lived to the age of 64. Goodwin asserts that alcohol fueled Faulkner's genius, allowing the shy and introspective man the confidence he needed to write (1990).

Charles Bukowski, who died at age 73, alluded to alcoholism, including his own, in the majority of his work. So much so that he was dubbed 'the Poet Laureate of Skid Row' and the recent collection of essays and reminiscences edited by Daniel Weizmann bears the title *Drinking with Bukowski* (2000). The poet's obsession fueled his poetry and provided most of his subject matter. Goodwin (1990) includes this verse from the poem *Who in the Hell is Tom Jones?* to exemplify Bukowski's numerous first-person vignettes of alcoholics:

I was drunk and in my
shorts. I tried to
separate them and fell,
wrenched my knee then
they were through the screen
door and down the walk
and out in the street.

Bukowski even had the audacity to appear in the movie *Ironweed*, portraying, of course, a drunk (Babenco, TAFT Entertainment Pictures, California). The stars Meryl Streep and Jack Nicholson, playing alcoholic lovers in New York during the 1930s, were nominated for Academy Awards. Charles Bukowski received no nomination: he simply played himself.

Substance abuse and women

In 1948, psychoanalyst Benjamin Karpman created a sensation in the lay press with his book *The Alcoholic Woman*, in which he claimed that, measured by any standard, female alcoholics tend to be sicker than alcoholic men: more depressed and anxious and exhibiting more abnormal personality traits. He also observed that many alcoholic women had alcoholic fathers. Certainly this is the case in the life of Susan Cheever, daughter of novelist John Cheever, as described in her book *Note Found in a Bottle: My Life as a Drinker* (1999). Karpman also observed that many alcoholic women ended their lives by suicide, an observation that seems valid still: Janis Joplin and Judy Garland, both substance abusers, actively committed suicide, while Marilyn Monroe 'accidentally' drank and drugged herself to death.

While men often brag about their alcohol and illicit drug use, few women do so, especially beyond college age. The fictional female detective who drinks excessively is rare, certainly when compared to her male counterpart. Social and cultural norms have placed a far greater stigma on female alcoholics and addicts, who are still often considered to be sexually promiscuous 'fallen women'. This societal judgmentalism has resulted in secret drinking on the part of many women; the hidden alcoholic, par excellence. As a consequence of 'closeting', mentioned earlier, women face a higher risk of progressing to advanced stages of alcoholism or other forms of chemical dependency before detection. Megan Moran's *Lost Years: Confessions of a Woman Alcoholic* (1985) deals frankly with both the secrecy and the shame indicated by her title: the absent life, the need to confess and the alienation.

Physician Martha Morrison includes similar themes in *White Rabbit* (1989). Morrison writes eloquently about her 17-year battle with alcoholism and her eventual recovery at a hospital, which specializes in the treatment of addicted physicians. In Morrison's words:

> Over an incredibly short time I developed true alcoholism with all the characteristics of the disease – the hidden bottles, the inability to stop, the denial. I didn't know I was an alcoholic, and of course nobody would accept that the fair-haired boy was drunk. Finally the drinking interfered with my work to such an extent that I was fired from Cox Hospital. Over the preceding three

years I had been hospitalized twenty-two times – never for alcoholism, of course – always for the flu, rectal bleeding, or for some other malady that actually resulted from drinking . . . . (Morrison 1989)

Dr Morrison took her recovery very seriously, even going to live with homeless people for three months. She describes this period where she slept under bridges, panhandled, and got to know her fellow 'bums' as a spiritual experience. Director Martin Scorsese, in his 1999 film *Bringing Out the Dead* (Scorsese, Paramount Pictures, California), also explores the problem of substance abuse among care-givers: Nicolas Cage plays a wounded healer, a paramedic who fights his demons of death, loss, and burn-out with alcohol, as do many of his cohorts on the night shift and even on the day shift. Filming at night, with the strobing of emergency lights slicing into shadows, Scorsese uses 'jiggling' shots to pull the viewer into a race up rickety stairs, a jaw-clenching ride through midnight streets, or the blur of dawn seen by fatigued, alcohol-fuzzed eyes through the grimy windows of a battered ambulance.

Scorsese portrays squalor and frenzy, curses and prayers, messy death and messy life. Carolyn Knapp, however, relates an entirely different situation. *Drinking: a love story* (Knapp, 1997) details the experience of a woman who loved everything about alcohol: 'I loved it from the very beginning . . . I loved the sounds of drink: the slide of the cork as it eased out the wine bottle, the distinct glug-glug of booze pouring out of a glass, the clatter of ice in a tumbler . . . the rituals, the camaraderie of drinking with others, the warming, melting feeling of ease and courage it gave me.' As a high-functioning alcoholic, Caroline Knapp never lost a job, never got derailed by a hangover, never experienced Skid Row; in fact, her history with alcohol had been quite pleasurable, a sort of family tie.

Knapp's father, a prominent psychoanalyst, could not easily hug or praise her, but he could and did introduce her to 'the hushed ritual of tall pitchers and lemon twists', later expanding the lessons to include good wine (especially Spanish sherry) and single-malt Scotch; Knapp herself always preferred wine to whiskey. Knapp's upper middle-class neighborhood, in fact, was 'awash with alcohol', starting in high school. Only years after her father's death did Knapp realize that he had been an alcoholic and that her retarded half-brother had been a victim of fetal alcohol syndrome.

In Knapp's words, alcohol '. . . made me less shy, less inhibited, it gave me a voice. . . . It turned me into a version of myself that felt more comfortable'. By her late 20s, Knapp had become a weekly newspaper columnist and a heavy drinker, imbibing each afternoon at a bar with co-workers and continuing through dinner and late evening. Director Betty Thomas's new film *28 Days* (Thomas, Columbia Pictures Corp., California) portrays a similar situation: Sandra Bullock plays newspaper columnist Gwen Cummings, a life-of-the-party, witty, functioning alcoholic who at first cannot admit her addiction but who finally undergoes an unfunny recovery. Like many 'closeted' alcoholics, Knapp 'maintained': no one at work seemed to suspect her. 'By whatever external measures we use, I was doing fine,' she asserts; 'the job stayed intact. The finances stayed intact.' Asked later (after her recovery) if she could identify a point at which the drinking ran out of control, Knapp acknowledges that it snowballed after her father was diagnosed with a brain tumor.

Spending nearly every evening with her alcoholic parents, she began belting straight from their numerous bottles and hiding other bottles in 'handy' places such as bathrooms. And she began making to herself the alcoholic's typical promise, exploring the substance abuser's premise, intoning the addict's mantra: '... I [am] only doing this because I can't tolerate this situation. I'll stop when this is over.' But of course, she did not.

For three more years, through the deaths of both parents and a couple of bad relationships, through several close calls (including almost dropping two children onto a sidewalk), through drunken drives on midnight streets, Knapp continued the downward spiral. The end of her active alcoholism was, compared to those years, 'undramatic': a bad party culminating in a bad fight, followed by '... the drive home with one eye closed to keep the double vision at bay. The whole humiliating, awful thing.' In 1994, Knapp entered a rehabilitation center; after completing inpatient treatment, she joined AA.

Knapp tells her story precisely because she does *not* fit society's image of the alcoholic: the thief, the drifter, the rioter, the writer in search of a Muse, 'the bum on the street, the wife-abusing tough guy, the falling-down neighborhood lush' totally lacking in hygiene. But, insists Knapp, she is/was the hidden alcoholic, the masquerader, the closeted one: '... the alcoholic most of us probably do know – and some of us may be .... The colleague who never misses the after-work drink. The niece who always brings an extra bottle of wine to dinner and never lets her glass go empty. The friend who makes those slurred late-night calls.'

And she states in clear, non-technical terms the emotional battles (aside from the often wrenching physical struggles) facing any substance abuser who desires to regain control of his/her life: 'The idea of giving up drinking is absolutely horrifying to an active alcoholic. I know it was for me ... I wept. I thought I would never have fun again; I would never have an intimate conversation. But it's so important to communicate that things really do get better, that it's liberating, not devastating. I have my life back.'

Literature reflects life: we write (and sing, act and film) what we know. The literature of popular culture reflects society's love/hate relationship with mind- and mood-altering substances, particularly with alcohol. Until concern for the waste and horror of addiction outweighs fascination with its 'adventure', the epidemic will rage on.

4

Understanding the whole person: developmental issues in the patient-centered approach to substance abuse

Jerome D Cook and Antonnette V Graham

Editor's introduction

Having explored issues of both the disease and illness experience of substance abuse in Chapters 1 and 3, we now turn our attention to the second component of patient-centered medicine, 'understanding the whole person'. Brown and Weston (1995) note that insights gained from seeking to understand the disease and the illness experience must be integrated with an understanding of the whole person. This involves understanding both the patient's position in the lifecycle and his or her life context. In this chapter we will focus on issues related to the patient's position in the lifecycle, looking at differences in presentation of this disorder in adolescence, adulthood and in the geriatric age group. By so doing, we hope to elucidate how substance abuse disorders may impede the patient's ability to accomplish the developmental tasks that need to be accomplished in each of these life stages, and how sensitivity to these issues can enhance both our understanding of the patient and our ability to find common ground and hence intervene effectively. In the process of looking at patients in various life stages we will also begin our exploration of the patient's life context, looking at how substance abuse is affected by the patient's gender and cultural background. Our study of patient context will conclude in the succeeding chapter, where we will look in depth at two other key areas of the patient's context: family and work.

An understanding of how developmental issues affect the presentation of the person with substance abuse is important to the individual practitioner. Development can be defined as the process of interaction between the individual and the environment that leads to successful adaptation and growth over time. The discussion of developmental issues, however, has often focused predominantly on the childhood years. With the arrival of Erikson's (1963) theory of psychosocial development, it has been recognized that healthy maturation involves a continual adaptation to the environment and resolution of developmental tasks throughout the lifespan. Within the substance abuse literature, discussion of developmental issues has predominantly focused on prevention issues in adolescence. The problem of substance abuse and dependency, however, can interfere with healthy adaptation across the lifecycle and represents a maladaptation that impairs further growth.

The aim of this chapter is to identify lifespan, gender, and cultural issues in addiction and how they may present to the healthcare provider in the context of a patient-centered approach to the treatment of substance abuse. Understanding this context enables the clinician to improve communication with the patient, to listen to their construction and narrative of their concerns, and to increase awareness of factors impinging upon the patient, including their family, social network and culture. All of these factors enter into the patient–clinician interaction. Case study presentations will highlight how context issues such as gender and cultural background present across the lifespan, helping us to come to an understanding of the whole person that will facilitate treatment and prevention of substance abuse disorders.

A common concern in the treatment of addictions is overcoming what colleagues in AA have identified as 'terminal uniqueness'. Khantzian and Mack (1989) have described this as pathological narcissism. Examples of this trait include 'the belief that they can take care of problems themselves, that they are self-sufficient, and that they are able to retain the necessary control over alcohol [and other drugs] as well as other areas of their lives' (Nace, 1997). Due to the insidious nature of substance dependency, it can often take years of regular use of the substance, especially alcohol, before symptoms of dependency appear. Consequently, individuals frequently develop their own theories regarding factors in the etiology and maintenance of their addiction. The individual with substance dependency may believe that addressing these hypothesized causes will 'cure the problem' and allow the individual to return to a 'safe' level of substance use. Furthermore, individuals may identify the problems caused by their addiction as the reasons for their use. These coping mechanisms serve to provide a justification for the individual's use of alcohol and attempt to deflect attention away from the use of alcohol (e.g. 'I don't drink alcohol, just beer').

An important role for the health professional involved in treating individuals with substance dependency is to understand the context and meaning ascribed to substance use, in order to establish trust and rapport in the therapeutic relationship. The establishment of this trust and rapport is necessary in order for the individual to assimilate information and direction from the clinician. Levin (1995) noted that 'patients presenting with alcohol problems demonstrate considerable commonality, and even if that commonality is the product of their drinking rather than its cause, the clinician must deal with it.' This conceptualization has a close relationship to the traditional disease model of addiction. Yet, to intervene effectively in this process, clinicians must be aware not only of the various stages of the disease, they must also have knowledge of the individual and his or her developmental phases, and how these components interact. Developmental models of addiction can be found in the writings of a number of authors (e.g. Brown, 1985, 1995; Prochaska and DiClemente, 1986).

The progressive nature of substance dependency was first proposed in detail by authors such as Jellinek (1946, 1952). Although the specifics of this progression have been disputed, the progressive nature of symptomatic presentation has been replicated (Pokorny and Kanas, 1980). Premature emphasis on disease, as opposed to the narrative of the disease as chronicled by the patient, is likely to lead to the phenomenon of reactance (Brehm, 1966). This is a sociopsychological theory that hypothesizes that attempts to limit choice and free will by proscribing a certain behavior will increase the attractiveness of the proscribed behavior. In addition to whatever reinforcing properties were initially inherent in the behavior, engaging in the behavior will now have the added value of demonstrating the free will of the individual. In order to overcome this phenomenon, the message from the clinician must be seen as important, relevant, salient, achievable and in the best interests of the patient. The 'stage change' or 'transtheoretical' model of addiction (Prochaska and DiClemente, 1986) outlines strategies to move clients from abuse to healthy recovery by eliciting self-motivational statements, as opposed to making demands upon the client (e.g. Miller and Rollnick, 1991). This model and techniques are discussed in a later chapter in this book.

The current chapter will examine substance abuse and dependence at three different points in the lifespan: adolescence, adulthood, and older adulthood. The two adult case studies will also highlight the impact of the context of gender and cultural background, as we look at substance abuse issues in women and in the African American context.

Adolescence

Personal historical and developmental variables contribute to a predisposition to substance abuse and dependency. The genetic heritability of alcohol abuse and dependency has a growing body of evidence which was explored in depth in Chapter 2 (Grove *et al.*, 1990; Murray and Clifford, 1983; Schuckit and Smith, 1996). In addition to genetic predisposition, adolescent substance use is also signficantly affected by the influence of peers and the mass media (Bandura, 1977). The family also plays a major role in evolving patterns of substance use, with important factors including permissive attitudes toward substance use by parents, parental substance use, the quality of the relationship between parents and children (Hird *et al.*, 1997), and access to alcohol and drugs at home (Resnick *et al.*, 1997).

Psychological changes which occur during adolescence include increased peer group influences, conformity and fear of rejection, changes in self-image and sexuality brought on by puberty, introspection, egocentrism, self-consciousness, risk-taking and sensation-seeking, perception of invulnerability, emphasis on immediate as opposed to long-term consequences, and affiliation with and acceptance by peers (Hird *et al.*, 1997). Peer use of alcohol is a particular risk factor for drinking in adolescents, and may be of even greater importance among teenage girls (Gomberg, 1998).

Adolescents with low self-esteem may be particularly susceptible to peer pressure to experiment with alcohol and drugs. Jones (1971) found that feelings of low self-esteem in teenage girls were predictive of drinking problems later in life. Adolescent girls who are receiving treatment for alcohol problems are more likely than boys to have a history of depression that predates their problems with alcohol (Deykin *et al.*, 1992). Likewise, heavy drinking and drug use provide a tempting avenue for risk-taking and sensation-seeking for some adolescents. The development of sexuality is influenced by substance use as well, and studies have indicated that alcohol consumption contributes both to an increase in sexual encounters and to higher levels of unsafe sexual practices by decreasing condom use (Strunin and Hingson, 1992). Heavy use of substances in adolescence may interfere with other stage-appropriate developmental tasks. Adolescents who abuse alcohol and drugs may have difficulty establishing their identity and successfully separating from parents.

As in adults, early signs of adolescent substance over-use are subtle and, because experimentation is common, are easily overlooked by parents and physicians. Screening for substance use problems, which is addressed in detail in Chapter 6, may be more difficult than in adults, since fewer physical signs exist and the history of use is shorter. Preventive guidelines for adolescent care include screening every adolescent for alcohol or drug use as a part of routine healthcare (Elster and Kunznets, 1994), with a goal of early detection and intervention.

Case study: the case of Patricia

The case of Patricia provides an example of how individual personal variables during adolescence are relevant to the presentation of the patient with substance abuse issues. Patricia Hathaway is a 17-year-old 11th grade student at a private high school. She is the youngest of three children and the only daughter. Her oldest brother is a fourth-year medical student at Johns Hopkins and her other brother is a pre-law student at Yale. Her father is a family physician and her mother is a senior partner in a law firm that her great grandfather established in the 1880s. Patricia's paternal grandfather is a cardiologist in Chicago. Over the last few years, Patricia has seen her physician several times for sports physicals, mild acne and menstrual cramps.

A week ago, she hit a tree while driving her mother's car. She was on her way home from visiting some 'new friends'. She had been taken to the local emergency room and treated for minor lacerations to her face and arms. Her blood alcohol level revealed that she had been drinking, but was not legally drunk. She was told to return to her primary care physician, Dr Elizabeth Johnson, to have the stitches removed. In the following interview, Dr Johnson, who is unaware of the accident, finds an opportunity for substance abuse intervention in the course of a 'routine suture removal.'

Dr J: 'Hi, Patricia. I see that you are here to have some stitches removed. What happened?'

Patricia: 'Oh, I just had a little accident.'

Dr Johnson remembers Patricia as being a bubbly, energetic teen but today she seems withdrawn and sad. She does not make eye contact. Dr Johnson decides to inquire about the feelings being expressed in her non-verbal behavior.

Dr J: You look upset.

Although Patricia's lower lip quivers a bit, she shakes her head. Dr Johnson knows there is something wrong and searches further for the unspoken concerns.

Dr J: Patricia, I've known you for many years and you seem different today. I'm concerned about you.

Patricia looks up and Dr Johnson sees tears forming in her eyes.

Dr J: Want to talk about what's happening?

Hesitant at first, Patricia tells Dr Johnson about the car accident.

Patricia: My parents are really upset and disappointed with me, like usual.

Dr J: What do you mean, like usual?

Patricia talks about feeling so inadequate compared to her two older brothers who are such superstars. She feels her parents would like her better if she were a boy. They often make comments about her 'being a moody adolescent girl'. She admits that she has felt sad for the last year, has lost interest in track (even though she was in the State finals the previous year), and that her grades are going down.

Many questions begin to rush through Dr Johnson's mind: Was Patricia drinking when she had the accident? How depressed is she? Is she using alcohol to medicate her sadness? Was the accident a suicide attempt?

Dr Johnson feels a twinge of guilt as she thinks about the limited time scheduled for this visit, but knows she has to explore the situation further.

Her questions reveal that Patricia is not suicidal, but is mildly depressed and that she was drinking when she had the accident. Questions about drinking reveal that Patricia has several new friends who drink a lot more than she does, and they frequently drink and drive. In addition, Patricia sometimes drinks alone and drinks to relieve tension. Recently, Patricia began to use marijuana. Patricia states that she doesn't think that her parents would be bothered by her drinking because they 'enjoy a few martinis' each evening and sometimes share with her. She is somewhat defensive about her marijuana use, again stating that it is not as much of a problem as her parents' drinking.

Dr Johnson explains that she is concerned about the sadness Patricia is feeling and is worried about her use of alcohol. She also expresses concern about the physical danger of drinking and driving, and asks Patricia to verbally contract with her not to do this again. Patricia agrees. Dr Johnson notes Patricia's comments about her parents' alcohol use, but decides not to explore that any further today. They agree upon a plan that includes some limits on what Dr Johnson will tell Mrs Hathaway, who is in the waiting room. Patricia agrees to talk to someone about her sadness and her use of alcohol and marijuana.

Tears run down Mrs Hathaway's face as she agrees that Patricia should be seen for an evaluation of her depression and alcohol and drug use.

Two weeks later, Patricia returns for a follow-up visit. Since the previous encounter, she has entered an outpatient adolescent treatment program and the family is engaged in the treatment program's family therapy component. Mrs Hathaway has decided that alcohol is probably a problem for her. She has begun to attend AA and has entered therapy to understand the impact on her of her own father's heavy drinking. Dr Hathaway is thinking about starting to go to Al-Anon.

The clinician's sensitivity to classic adolescent lifecycle issues helped make this a life-changing clinical encounter for Patricia. The patient's drinking began in the context of both a positive family history (genetic predisposition) and parental permissiveness regarding substance use. Her new friendship with peers who drink and use drugs appears also to have contributed to her increasing use of psychoactive substances, including marijuana. The overall presentation of a change in friends, declining school performance, loss of interest in other activities and an episode of alcohol-related trauma included numerous classic features of adolescent substance abuse. Her comments to Dr Johnson regarding her feelings of inadequacy revealed both low self-esteem and signs of adolescent depression which may have preceded her substance abuse. Dr Johnson, sensitive to explore the origins and meaning of trauma in an adolescent patient, quickly found common ground with Patricia and turned a 'routine office visit' into an effective intervention for both the patient and her family.

Women in adulthood

In understanding substance abuse issues among women, it is important to understand differences in development that may influence their presentation. Clinicians may have a tendency to underestimate the importance of assessing and treating substance use problems in women, often believing that substance abuse disorders are primarily a male problem. As noted in Chapter 1, while both alcoholism prevalence (Grant, 1997b) and use of illegal drugs (USDHHS, 1998) are significantly less common in women than in men, the gap between male and female substance abuse appears to be narrowing. Recent data reporting equal use of alcohol, tobacco and other drugs among teenage boys and girls and increased binge drinking among female college students suggest that peer influences and conformity may be special problems for women. Tension between social pressures, parental pressures and societal pressures may lead to more secretive substance use among adolescent females, a trend that often continues into adulthood.

Recent data regarding genetic influences indicate that genetic factors exert a more modest influence in the expression of alcohol problems in women than in men (Kendler *et al.*, 1992; McGue *et al.*, 1992; Pickens *et al.*, 1991), and that environmental factors exert a greater influence. Younger women (aged 21–34) are more apt to engage in binge drinking and to drink away from home, which leads to auto accidents, problems with authorities and vulnerability to assaults. Increased drinking has been reported among working women, apparently due to increased availability of alcohol rather than the stress of multiple responsibilities. Marital status is clearly correlated with alcohol use. While married women's drinking patterns often tend to mirror those of their spouses, co-habiting women and divorced women report significantly higher rates of drinking and drinking problems (Wilsnack, 1996; Wilsnack *et al.*, 1991).

For many women who drink more heavily in early adulthood, this heavy drinking remits over time. However, between the ages of 35 and 49, some women develop chronic, persistent problems with symptoms of dependency. The result in many cases is the development of significant medical complications, which may begin earlier than in men and be more severe (Ashley *et al.*, 1977). Divorce, separation and children leaving home are frequent outcomes as well (Wilsnack, 1996).

Psychiatric complaints are significantly more frequent in substance-abusing women than in their male counterparts. The most common psychiatric diagnoses in women are depression and anxiety, as opposed to anti-social personality in men (Regier *et al.*, 1990). Psychotropic drugs are frequently prescribed to substance-abusing women, and are more likely to be misused by women than by men (Amodei *et al.*, 1996). Physicians frequently identify depression or anxiety as a primary diagnosis and do not identify these mental health problems as symptoms of an underlying substance abuse disorder. Physicians are more likely to refer a woman to a mental health provider or to treat her pharmacologically than to screen for alcohol and drug abuse and initiate substance abuse treatment. Older women's increased use of psychotropic medications also predisposes them to other problems related to interactions between alcohol and drugs. Since metabolism of drugs slows with age, interaction with alcohol can occur several days after taking the medication.

Pregnancy does not offer protection against the attraction of cigarettes, alcohol or drugs. As highlighted with the case of Lakeisha in Chapter 1, the shame associated with substance use during pregnancy and the fear, especially among low income women, of having their child placed in foster care makes identification more difficult. Alcohol use during pregnancy is the leading cause of preventable mental retardation, and smoking contributes to profound increases in infant morbidity and mortality. Judgmental, moralistic and punitive attitudes on the part of healthcare providers may significantly impede effective identification and treatment. In order to be effective in managing substance abuse problems among women, clinicians and treatment centers must give special attention to issues such as women's only groups, care during pregnancy, and childcare. These focused and supportive interventions improve the access to substance abuse treatment, and are thus likely to be more effective.

The correlation between substance abuse and STDs was addressed in the previous section on adolescence. Substance abuse problems in women are also correlated with victimization (Liebschutz *et al.*, 1997). A high percentage of women who seek treatment for addictions reveal a history of sexual or physical abuse (Kendler *et al.*, 2000) . Also, women who have been drinking are more likely to be victims of rape or physical assault than non-drinking women or men. Victimization in women with substance abuse problems is related to increased utilization of medical care and clinicians should be urged to avoid a 'blame the victim ' mindset (Liebschutz *et al.*, 1997).

Because of the stigma associated with substance use problems in women, questions need to be presented in a non-threatening, empathetic manner. When significant abuse or shame issues are present, the caregiver may need to gather information slowly over a series of office visits, using the continuity experience to develop the trust level necessary to explore these painful issues. Through the use of both verbal and non-verbal cues, the clinician must demonstrate respect and affirm the patient's dignity, giving her opportunity to share her illness experience and to be fully understood as a whole person and as a valued individual. The following case illustrates the importance of gender issues in the presentation and recovery of an adult female patient.

Case study: the case of Jean S
Jean S is a 37-year-old female of German descent. She is divorced from her first husband, who has custody of her two children, aged 11 and 13. They

live in another State with their father and stepmother. Jean recently moved to the South-west from the industrial North-east with her fiancé of one year, due to a job opportunity for him. She now presents because she has relapsed to alcohol, cocaine and amphetamine use and is profoundly depressed. She reports using six to 12 beers daily despite previous attempts at sobriety. She is taking Prozac (fluoxetine) that was prescribed for her during a previous treatment period one year ago. She used $200 of cocaine on three days during the past month and used amphetamines from a friend when the cocaine ran out. Recently, she has been contemplating suicide due to guilt over her relapse and fear of its impact on her current relationship. Jean experienced severe guilt over her divorce and loss of custody due to her addictions, and experienced anger over the refusal of her children's father and stepmother to forward mail to her children or allow phone contact.

Aware of the extreme shame and guilt that Jean is experiencing, her family physician devotes much of the interview to empathic listening and suggests immediate referral to a substance abuse treatment center. Jean complies and is enrolled in an intensive outpatient treatment program which addresses both her substance dependency and depression. After four weeks she returns, reporting that she has become pregnant. She expresses concern about continuing to take Prozac, but is encouraged to continue this due to the greater risk posed by her relapse to drugs and alcohol if her depression should recur.

As therapy continues, Jean develops pregnancy complications, making it difficult to keep weekly outpatient appointments and she discontinues treatment. Six weeks after the birth of her baby she calls, tearfully indicating that she feels anxious, stressed and depressed. She feels guilty about feeling this way, stating that she knows she should feel grateful for her recent marriage to her fiancé, the birth of a healthy baby and having maintained her sobriety. Nonetheless, she reports that following the birth of her baby she began to experience severe depression, fear and guilt; fear that she might relapse and guilt that she felt depressed despite having a supportive husband and a new baby. Her thoughts were reflective of negative thinking typical of depression, including fears that she was overweight from the birth and that her husband would leave her. She experienced guilt over feeling too tired and stressed to keep her house cleaned and straightened. She felt that she was a poor mother, wife and person.

Her physician, aware of the need to address both substance abuse issues and post-partum depression, continued her pharmacotherapy, focused on identifying and countering self-defeating beliefs, and assisted her in clarifying the need to remain committed to sobriety as her first priority. As Jean herself identified her sense of feeling overwhelmed by all the responsibilities of motherhood, she worked with her physician to produce a plan which included taking time to go to therapy and taking brief, periodic 'stress breaks' during the day. In addition, she made plans to communicate both her needs and her plan of action to her husband and get his support, and to counter feelings of guilt by verbally affirming herself for taking time for self-care behaviors.

Adult development in an African American context

The past two decades have witnessed the rise and, hopefully, the beginning of the fall of the cocaine, and particularly the crack cocaine, epidemic. Unfortunately, however, the MTF studies of high school students have recently shown a slow but steady rise in annual and monthly use of cocaine and crack cocaine since the early 1990s. According to the National Household Survey (NHS), adult African American males (26 years and older) have been particularly vulnerable to the cocaine and crack epidemic, using at twice the rate of Whites and Hispanics. This represents a reversal of the pattern in adolescence and young adulthood (aged 12–25), where Whites and Hispanics report using at two to three times the rate of same-age African Americans (USDHHS, 1998). Sociological explanations of this reversal have yet to be fully articulated. In the African American culture, the roles of extended family, the church and awareness of cultural history have been hypothesized to be protective factors against substance abuse. A significant risk factor, however, is the role of poverty (Rouse, 1989). Surveys have indicated that adult African American males are more likely to be users of illicit drugs, particularly cocaine, and that this is particularly true for unemployed or impoverished males. The rates of unemployment or poverty in the African American community thus present special risks.

An early study of African American males aged 30–35 found that growing up fatherless was a predictor of drug use in this population (Robins and Murphy, 1967). One striking consequence of the use of dangerous drugs is the high rate of drug-related deaths in hospital emergency rooms among male African Americans, with the majority of deaths occurring at ages 30–39 (Rouse, 1989).

A particular strength among African American families is their strong religious orientation and the deep religious commitment of their members. Nobles (1972) traces the roots of the centrality of religion and its relationship to community to pre-slavery West Africa. He notes that many African languages did not have a specific word for religion, as 'religion was such an integral part of man's existence that it and he were inseparable'.

Despite the continued presence of racist attitudes and barriers in the US military, as in mainstream culture, the military culture has traditionally been a route to equality of opportunity, achievement, education and training for African Americans. The military environment has been noted to provide structure in addition to opportunity, but also a culture where peer influence dominates and of which substance abuse can become a part (Kutz, 1996). As the patient-centered clinician deals with individual patients, it is important to examine all sources of cultural variation, from religious and ethnic differences to gender, sexual orientation, disability and veteran status.

The developmental tasks of young adulthood and adulthood involve resolving the conflicts of intimacy vs isolation and generativity vs stagnation (Erikson, 1963), often focused around the resolution of the difference between an individual's dreams and aspirations and his or her actual accomplishments (Brown and Tooley, 1989). As Rosenberg and Farrell (1976) have observed, these are difficult tasks for many individuals, resulting in increases in substance abuse, divorce and suicide during the midlife years. The following case study reveals how a substance abuse disorder develops in the life of an African American male seeking to deal with these lifecycle issues.

Case study: the case of William J

William J is a 43-year-old African American male who presented requesting substance abuse treatment for cocaine dependency. During the previous year, the patient had separated from his wife of 20 years. She had taken out a restraining order against him after being assaulted by him following a cocaine binge, for which he was currently serving probation. They had been high school sweethearts who married after his military service. They have two children, ages nine and 15. In the past year, the patient had been terminated after 18 years in a well-paid job in the transportation industry due to a second positive urine drug screen for cocaine.

As a child, the patient had been cared for by his maternal grandparents and mother after the father had abandoned the family. He was the younger of two children. He had been introduced to drugs and alcohol in the military, but had been sober since shortly before his marriage until two years ago. In his early adult life, the patient had successfully accomplished the tasks of developing intimate relationships and raising a family. Following success in the military, he had worked for 18 years in a productive and well-paying position of responsibility in the transportation industry.

Despite achieving these milestones, he experienced a 'midlife crisis' during which he began to doubt the significance of these accomplishments and threatened them through his use of cocaine. He described in graphic terms his internal struggles to reconcile his accomplishments with the dreams he had had for his own life, a conflict which Brown and Tooley (1989) describe as the major crisis of adulthood. In the midst of this crisis, he reunited with an old football team mate from high school, who had earlier introduced him to crack cocaine. Prior to that time, he had been active in church and family activities. He quickly became addicted, using over $800 worth of cocaine each weekend, helping his friend distribute the cocaine and having extramarital and unprotected sex.

On two occasions, his cocaine use was detected on a routine drug screen on the job, and he was terminated. He reported a good deal of resentment toward his employer, noting that a co-worker had not been fired, despite an arrest for aggravated assault, while he had been fired for his positive drug screen. The fact that his co-worker was White added a racial component to his animosity toward his employer. In addition, his seniority on the job contributed to his resentment and feeling of being persecuted.

The patient also experienced marital and family conflict as his usage and spending increased. He became more agitated and abusive in relationships with both his wife and children. Despite his own behavior, the patient continued to display resentment toward his wife, believing that she should continue to support him because of their marriage vows. Nonetheless, it was his desire to be reunited with his wife and children that motivated him to seek help for his cocaine addiction.

The clinician began by seeking to understand the patient in the context of his cultural context, his family setting, and the critical lifecycle issues he was facing. He began by not only recording the details of the patient's cocaine use and its associated consequences, but also eliciting his ideas, expectations and feelings about his cocaine use, as well as his observations on its effect on his life. The clinician faced the challenge of remaining sensitive to the patient's perceptions of victimization as an African American, based on the reality of unfair treatment in the past and present, while at the same time avoiding colluding with the patient in rationalizing harmful actions. As he explored the context of the peer relationship that led to William's substance use, he discovered a high level of dependency on affirmation by his peers and a pattern of overt masculine behaviors that is typical of males from father-absent homes (Brown and Tooley, 1989). As treatment progressed and William gained an understanding of the pharmacological and psychological consequences of chronic and heavy cocaine use, he was able to identify how the cocaine fed his own grandiosity and need to be the center of attention. He was able to acknowledge the increase in paranoia and persecutory ideas following cocaine use. He was also able to identify how the cocaine use may have been exaggerating pre-existing narcissistic tendencies arising out of the emotional hurt and compensation for the abandonment of his father over 40 years ago.

Most importantly, he began to recognize the feelings and values behind his strong motivation to reunite with his wife and children. The patient expressed a deep sense of failure in his roles as husband, father, and breadwinner. Having grown up in a single-parent family, he had never been part of a family where he had observed a positive male role model in these tasks.

He had grown up in a culture of males in football, the military, and the railroad industry that emphasized physical prowess, dominance, winning and masculine interests. Despite benefiting from many positive aspects of this culture, he lacked a male role model who resolved the conflict of intimacy in a domestic setting. Nonetheless, he described almost 20 years of deeply satisfying relationships with his wife and children prior to his cocaine dependency. His involvement in church activities during that period had reinforced and strengthened his dedication to his family, and had resulted in a personal spiritual faith that was extremely meaningful to him. Both his commitment to his family and his spiritual life had suffered greatly during his period of cocaine dependency.

As treatment progressed, the clinician helped William to validate the genuine accomplishments of his early adult years and to crystallize the maturation of his own value system, in which caring and providing for his family played a central role. His church played a key role in his recovery process, as it has for many in the African American culture (Hudson, 1986; Knox, 1986), helping him maintain his sobriety, as well as helping him to come to peace with his midlife issues.

Alcohol abuse among older adults

The elderly are the age group at lowest risk from alcohol and illicit drug problems. Proposed reasons for this fact include self-imposed limitations on consumption due to a decreased ability to detoxify alcohol and other drugs, decreased consumption by individuals in recovery from earlier problems related to alcohol and drugs, and fear of interactions with prescription medications. The elderly do use and at times abuse large quantities of both prescription and over-the-counter medications, and clinicians must obtain careful histories to determine exactly what substances an individual patient is taking. Substance abuse problems, when present, are often overlooked and underdiagnosed. Clinicians' index of suspicion regarding alcohol-related problems, for example, is often low (Zimberg, 1995), and signs of alcohol abuse or dependency typically seen in younger patients may be absent. An older person who is retired, does not own a car, has few family or social contacts and has few responsibilities outside the home may report few alcohol-related problems due to the change in roles related to aging (Graham, 1986). Instead, housing problems, social isolation, lack of self-care and poor nutrition may be indicators of problems associated with substance abuse. Medical complications, such as changes in red blood cell indices which are easily detected on the hemogram, may actually be more frequent in the elderly, who appear to be more physiologically vulnerable (Hunt *et al.*, 1988). Nonetheless, substance abuse-related symptoms and abnormal laboratory tests may be less easily differentiated from the effects of other chronic illnesses and from side effects of medications.

In late-onset alcoholism, increased alcohol use and abuse follow one or more events perceived by the individual as significant losses. Such losses may include retirement, loss of physical health, death and illness of friends and family, social isolation, financial problems, and physical and cognitive declines that lead to barriers and inactivity.

Erikson (1963) has written that the main developmental conflict among those over 65 years of age is one of 'ego integrity' vs despair. When successfully negotiated, individuals are able to look back over their lives and feel that they have been true to their sense of self, and have achieved a personal definition of success. Although not empirically investigated, the rising rate of completed suicide with increasing age (Vaillant and Blumenthal, 1990) argues that resolution of this stage is one of the more difficult life tasks. Depression, alcoholism and dementia are the most common diagnostic groups among the elderly who complete suicide (Bongar, 1991). An important consideration in this regard is the effect of substance abuse on individuals' ability to deal with the interpersonal losses and conflicts common in this age group. One study reported that loss and conflict events were more likely to precipitate suicide among alcoholics, whether or not they were depressed, than was the case with non-abusing depressed patients (Rich *et al.*, 1988). This likely reflects the increased impulsivity and decreased inhibition associated with alcohol abuse.

The following case example demonstrates how the patient-centered approach can be used to engage and address the losses and changes in roles which are often key components of this disorder in the elderly.

Case study: the case of Bob M

Bob M is a 60-year-old Caucasian male from a rural Appalachian mountain community. He is divorced twice. Following his second divorce 10 years ago, he was hospitalized for a suicide attempt via overdose of Xanax (alprazolam). Two years ago, following the death of his mother in a nursing home, where she had been treated for Alzheimer's disease, the patient moved in to take care of his ailing and elderly father, giving up his job as a hardware salesman. He supported himself through part-time work and his father's social security check. His father died at age 78. Three months later the patient, who had never sought treatment for alcohol problems, was ordered to enter treatment by the court because of driving under the influence of alcohol. In his will, the father had not specified maintaining the residence intact, but instead requested that his estate be equally divided among the patient and his two siblings. A sister stated her intention to have the residence sold with the profits split among the three children, and informed her brother that he would have to leave within the ensuing three months. Thus within two years, the patient lost his mother and father, his job, his roommate and only regular social contact and his home, and was at odds with his only surviving family members. In addition, these losses were reminiscent of his two prior divorces. Due to his heavy drinking for the past 20 years, Bob's health was deteriorating. Giving up alcohol, the one object that had 'always been there' for him, was a frightening thought for Bob. The following therapeutic exchange demonstrates how patient-centered dialogue helped him acknowledge his ambivalence regarding his alcohol use and the depth of his recent losses.

Bob: I don't know what to do! I've lost everything!

Interviewer: You've been through a lot recently. Tell me about one of the things you've lost.

The interviewer's first statement is an example of reflective listening. The second statement is an open-ended one designed to elicit the patient's narrative. The phrasing that asks for one loss allows the patient to attempt to focus his distress and improve his articulation of it, while potentially providing the interviewer with information about what the patient perceives as the major problem. It may also serve as a 'foot-in-the-door' technique, such that once the patient articulates what he considers to be his main problem, he may also choose to continue voicing additional concerns.

Bob: I don't have a home! They're taking it away from me.

Interviewer: Who are they?

Bob: My sister. She's selling the house. She's told me I need to leave within three months. I took care of our dad for two years and now I'm not going to have a place to live.

The patient's response reflects the fear of loss of shelter and safety that one might expect to be primary according to a hierarchy of needs (Maslow, 1968). Instead of expressing statements reflecting 'ego integrity' as Erikson might wish for in the case of healthy maturational development, he communicates a tone of despair, perhaps due to previous developmental failures. He also stays away from the emotion of depression that may rise from the loss of family through death and estrangement that threaten needs of belonging. Instead of depression, the first emotions evident appear to be anger and a feeling of persecution. Direct questions regarding alcohol use at this point might exaggerate these emotions and harm therapeutic rapport.

Interviewer: It's hard to begin making plans while you're still grieving.

This statement offers an interpretation that also provides an opportunity for the patient to articulate emotions beyond anger. It also acknowledges that grief may be on-going or long-lasting. Although the interviewer's main concern may be the patient's alcohol use, he first responds to the patient's need to have his grief and loss recognized and validated.

Bob: Yeah, I don't know what I'm going to do.

Interviewer: What other concerns do you have?

The patient does not accept the opportunity now to express grief or other emotions in this context, or may not have the ability to do so. Feeling it is too early in the therapeutic relationship to offer direct advice, the interviewer chooses to seek further definition of the scope of the problems facing the patient by offering an open-ended question. The change in topic, rather than a reflective comment, broadens the scope and avoids reinforcing the helplessness evident in Bob's last sentence.

Bob: I've just been feeling sick and tired.

Interviewer: How so?

Bob: My stomach's been acting up and my nerves have gone bad.

This question allows the patient to elaborate on physical symptoms. The elderly may tend to focus on these more concrete symptoms rather than depression or alcohol use. This patient's description of his physical symptoms also fits a cultural norm that tends to emphasize somatic complaints without a specified etiology, with a style of expression that almost gives the physical system a mind of its own. It is important to pay attention to physical symptoms that may be exacerbated by alcohol use. These can be used later in feedback to the patient about the relationship of alcohol to these symptoms for motivational purposes.

By this time, rapport has been established, and it may be appropriate to ask about substance habits, beginning with potentially less threatening discussions of caffeine and nicotine, followed by alcohol and other drugs. In this case, the CAGE questions (described in detail in Chapter 6) were employed, providing useful factual information on consequences of the patient's use as well as providing the opportunity for him to discuss his perceptions of his use. The Geriatric Depression Scale (GDS), a validated, standardized instrument used to screen for depression in the elderly, was also employed. His answers revealed moderate to severe depression and several signs of alcohol dependency. At this time, the interviewer chose to provide a summary of problems identified by the patient, present the diagnosis and begin to work toward finding common ground upon which to make a treatment plan.

Interviewer: Well, you certainly have been through the wringer lately. The loss of one's father is one of the most significant events that men endure.

This beginning statement acknowledges the theme of loss reflected in all of the events Bob has been experiencing. It avoids stigmatizing him with the label 'alcoholic'. Although it may be desirable for him to eventually accept this label through involvement in AA, the label is not a medical term and the interviewer chooses to allow the patient to accept or reject it in his own time, rather than imposing it as a diagnosis. In addition, the statement begins to normalize the events and the grieving process, and implies eventual resolution and endurance.

Interviewer (cont.): And I'm sure it hasn't helped to have the family arguing during this time.

This statement acknowledges the problem without choosing sides.

Interviewer (cont.): It sounds like you've been concerned about your use of alcohol during this time, and it's been another part of your life that's been out of control, to the point of breaking the law and risking your life and others. It also appears that some of the physical symptoms you're experiencing are the result of your alcohol use, and you've become physically and emotionally dependent on the alcohol.

In order to start working on these problems, you'll need to be mentally and physically free of the effects of alcohol. We can help you get to that point so that you can begin to reorder your life, and you'll need to have as much support in that as possible. We'll have a social worker talk to you about housing options, and is there a pastor or chaplain you'd like to speak with?

The clinician engaged Bob by identifying and validating his sense of loss and seeking common ground around the theme of rebuilding his life. Intervention focused on addressing Bob's multiple needs to help re-establish independence. A social worker helped him locate long-term housing while he stayed at a domiciliary during treatment. He discussed options for returning to work as a salesman. Through contact with a local church, he was encouraged to reconnect to previously neglected spiritual beliefs, as well as to understand the process of grief. His use of AA as a support group helped him to meet socialization needs as well as focusing him on the priority of sobriety. Intervention also addressed symptoms of depression that occurred with his alcohol dependency, bereavement and the stress of the sudden role changes. The emphasis on all of the patient's needs, understanding the alcohol use in context, and the clinician's holistic, respectful approach built a solid patient–clinician relationship which enabled the patient to perceive that the goal of treatment was his improved overall well-being, and not simply the removal of a vice. Thus, the healthcare provider could be seen as helping to provide something positive, rather than adding to his losses by threatening to take something away.

Conclusion

A patient-centered approach to the treatment of substance abuse must view the patient not through the prism of diagnostic labeling and the stigma society associates with such labels, but through an understanding of the whole person and his or her use of addictive substances in context of his or her age, gender and sociocultural background. A patient-centered approach to treatment will acknowledge both the strong reinforcing properties of the substances and the devastating consequences of excessive use of these substances upon the life of the individual patient. The recognition that the substance is responsible for both of these effects will assist the healthcare provider in identifying ambivalence and points of resistance to change.

A thorough history and allowing the patient time and comfort in expressing the full range of problems and symptoms will facilitate the most accurate assessment. Even when the patient is suspected of minimizing use and consequences of use, a patient-centered approach to interviewing will help to identify factors that may be influencing such minimization.

The most important aspect of the patient-centered approach is the development of the therapeutic rapport and trust, which often may have been missing in the lives of substance-abusing patients. Such an approach recognizes the limits of attempting to control or change a person's behavior, and instead focuses on making changes identified as important by the patient. The ability to understand the patient in the context of age, gender, ethnicity, religion, geographic origins, personality development, class or any other relevant variable will assist the healthcare provider in understanding the meaning that the patient associates with his or her substance use. By understanding this context, he or she is more likely to be in a position to add something of value to the patient's life and to be a coach and collaborator in the process of change, as opposed to being seen as another obstacle or demand upon the patient's resources.

While emphasizing the value of a patient-centered approach to substance abuse treatment and, particularly, emphasizing the value of a holistic approach to the patient, it is important to take into account limitations of this approach. The patient-centered approach recognizes the free will of the patient, and that the patient may initially have conflicting goals, timelines and expectations of treatment process and outcome. This may be particularly difficult for close family, friends and even other treatment professionals to accept. In such cases, Al-Anon or Nar-Anon, for friends and family of people with substance dependency, may help to acknowledge powerlessness and loss of control over others' substance use behaviors, and redirect their energy toward making positive changes in their own lives. In addition, employers, agencies, insurance and managed-care companies may have agendas different from the patient and the clinician. As S Brown (1995) notes, 'a single-minded focus on quick behavioral change runs the risk of unwittingly trapping the therapist in the same double-bind struggle as the alcoholic and those close to the drinker'. In this context, she notes, 'rarely is the treatment related to the client's time frame, needs, wishes, or conflicts that might be quite amenable to exploration within the framework of an unfolding therapeutic relationship backed up by a long-term developmental model of change'. The patient-centered approach works by identifying the patient's own definition of the problem as well as the goals of treatment through a 'collaborative conversation about behavior changes' (Rollnick *et al.*, 1999) to find common ground.

The rewards of a patient-centered approach to substance abuse treatment include becoming a part of the human journey toward change through both successes and failures, in a way that acknowledges the dignity and worth of each individual.

5

Impact of substance abuse on the family and work

Sylvia Shellenberger and Gregory Phelps

Editor's introduction

The second of two chapters dealing with the second component of patient-centered medicine, 'understanding the whole person', this section focuses on two key areas of the patient's life context: the family and the work environment. In healthy families, as individuals are connected biologically, emotionally or legally within the family unit, they create a nurturing, safe and continuous environment which serves to promote the physical, psychological and social well-being of its members (Brown and Weston, 1995). Substance abuse often results in a dysfunctional family unit which is unsafe and emotionally destructive and erodes the physical and psychological well-being of its members. Indeed, the dysfunctional patterns of co-dependency and enabling were first recognized and defined through the study of substance-abusing families. While much of the research cited in this chapter was done with alcoholic families, the findings are also typical of families affected by abuse of virtually all kinds of psychoactive substances. Substance abuse may present in the primary care setting due to physical or emotional consequences in either the patient or another family member who is trying to survive in this dysfunctional family system. Thus, it is essential that the patient-centered clinician understands the full impact of this disease on the family system and is prepared to recognize it and inter-vene. The work environment, another key part of the system in which most patients function, assumes an extremely high level of importance for the substance abuser. Because substance-abusing patients frequently experience negative consequences of their disease on the job, which is necessary for their day-to-day survival, the work environment provides a key opportunity for disease recognition and a powerful moti-vator toward recovery. In this chapter, Drs Shellenberger and Phelps pro-vide us with an in-depth analysis of how the patient-centered clinician can better understand the substance-abusing patient as a whole person by gaining insight into his or her family and work situation and use these insights to facilitate diag-nosis and recovery.

Case study: a true story
My waitress at breakfast yesterday arrived at our two-some table smiling, but my colleague on the other side of the table glanced up and stifled a gasp. 'What?' I asked puzzled. By way of explanation the waitress turned full face to me, showing the bruising on her forehead and shiner around her right eye. 'My husband', she explained, 'or rather my ex-husband. Got liquored up last night and came over to "smooth" things over. Hell', she continued matter of factly, 'Drinkin's why I threw him out in the first place. I just got out of the emergency room this morning in time to be docked for being late to my shift here.'

It is a medical rarity that alcoholic patients arrive at the doors of their healthcare provider understanding their diagnosis. Much like patients with syphilis, the last century's 'great pretender', most patients affected by alcoholism present to professionals with symptoms of insomnia, agitation, depression or sexual difficulties. More dramatically, they may present with broken bones from accidents or falls. Medical problems might include acute GI hemorrhage, neuropathies related to alcohol poisoning or seizures related to withdrawal. In the workplace, substance abuse may present as industrial accidents, chronic tardiness, decreasing productivity or failed drug tests.

Family members of the alcoholic surface with symptoms as well. Spouses of alcoholics disclose headaches, sleeplessness, abdominal distress or inability to find any joy in life. Children of alcoholics present with symptoms of school problems, abdominal pain or temper tantrums. Adult children of alcoholics complain of nightmares, flashbacks, difficulty concentrating, overcommitments from enabling behavior or sleeping too much. These are signals to the primary care practitioner that the problems of alcohol have pervaded and taken their toll on the family system. Thick medical charts reveal diagnoses of liver failure, hypertension and gastritis in the alcoholic, chronic dysthymia and acute stress disorder in the spouse of the alcoholic, conduct disorder in children and post-traumatic stress disorder in adult children of alcoholics. Even more severe problems of family violence and child abuse, delinquency and drug use are not uncommon. The memories of trauma haunt family members for generations. Practitioners who take into account the pervasive nature of this problem by assessing and intervening with the family will have the greatest opportunity for influencing the family system.

As described in Chapter 4, the context of the problem of substance abuse with all of its layers of complexity needs to be understood by the healthcare providers. This chapter describes the context of the problem in two arenas: the family and work. Health promoting and dysfunctional family and work patterns are described, as well as ways of assessing the family and work situations. The goal of the chapter is to promote an attitude of curiosity on the part of the healthcare providers toward discovering the family and work influences that have brought the addicted patient or family to the door of the caregiver. With this attitude, the caregiver will be positioned to intervene with the patient and family demonstrating a spirit of collaboration, compassion and respect.

Subtance abuse is a family systems problem (Berenson 1976; Steinglass *et al.*, 1987). Like a Calder mobile, the family has its own stability and equilibrium – touch any part of the mobile and all parts swing to a new position in the overall sculpture. Substance abuse, when present, may become the central and organizing aspect of the mobile. The family organizes itself and establishes equilibrium around the substance abuse. Substance abuse compromises the health of the individual and has reverberations through all aspects of the patient's life, including the family and work setting. The healthcare provider is touched by the substance-abusing patient's compromised health status and has the potential of touching the patient in health-promoting ways so that the mobile swings in positive directions. Generations past and future as well as the extended family are often affected by the problem of alcoholism and substance abuse and can be resources to help effect change in the pattern of alcohol and drug use. The case of Juan Espinosa illustrates how one touch to the mobile creates a new sculpture. The genogram of Juan's family shows the pervasiveness of the problem of alcoholism throughout the family system.

Case study
Juan Espinosa, a 35-year-old Hispanic male, moved to a city in Southeastern US to take a position as supervisor of mechanics for a large garment

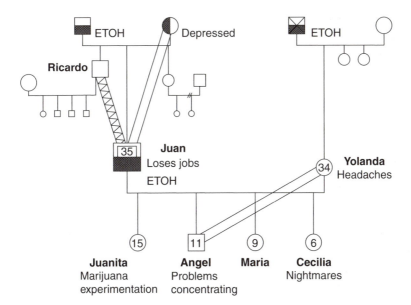

Figure 5.1   The Espinosa family.

manufacturing facility. A few months after his arrival, he suffered a minor injury that sent him to the doctor's office as part of a worker's compensation. Under the laws of the State in which he was working, he was also required to submit to a urine drug test and a breath alcohol test. The results were reported from the lab to the Medical Review Officer (i.e. a physician knowledgeable in substance abuse) as positive for marijuana and alcohol. The Medical Review Officer called the contact phone number that turned out to be Mr Espinosa's home. A woman answered who identified herself as Mrs Yolanda Espinosa. She said that Mr Espinosa was at work. She was asked to have her husband call the doctor's office. Mr Espinosa called back shortly, expressed surprise at the result, but offered no alternative explanation. He declined referral for counseling and hung up the telephone. The next day Mrs Espinosa called to say that her husband was about to lose his job 'again'. She was distraught at moving to what was to be a 'new chance' and asked about the counseling mentioned to her husband. She said her children became very upset wondering if they would have to move once again.

The reactions in the Espinosa family members are similar to those of other families affected by substance abuse. In the identified patient, there is often denial that substance abuse is a problem. In the spouse, after years of coping with the substance abuse, there are often feelings of anger, disillusionment, and resentment. Children react with fear when parents are arguing, disappointment because their alcoholic parent is repeatedly unavailable and culpability because many parental arguments are about the children. At the same time, children may experience a sense of unreality related to clearly abnormal, drug-induced behavior that is relabeled by an influential parent in denial as 'nothing'. Most often the patient in the family that presents to the healthcare provider is not the substance abuser but a spouse or child who becomes the designated patient. It is small wonder that the first 12-step program to form after the original AA was that of Al-anon, for families of alcoholics.

Family patterns

With substance abuse at the center of their lives, families cope the best they know how. Sometimes there are maladaptive roles and patterns. Roles in the family may become unbalanced and static. Sometimes families act in ways that are counterintuitive to what would be expected; that is, they may engage in patterns contributing to family dysfunction and even to continuance of the abuse. Typical maladaptive patterns seen in families include denial, rescuing and enabling, blaming, enmeshment, alienation, depression and stress-related symptoms, acting-out, punishing behaviors, lifecycle stagnation and violence. These roles and patterns may define the interactions within the family long after the departure or recovery of the chemically dependent member. Most families affected by substance abuse also show areas of great resilience and strength. The extended Espinosa family experienced all of these patterns; each of them is described here.

Denial

Family members and the abusers themselves often deny the existence or extent of a problem. In thinking about their own use, abusers minimize the amounts and frequency of their use. Many abusers believe that they can cut down or quit on their own whenever they want to. They believe occasional overuse of substances is not hurting anybody. In actuality, we know that many are hurt. Children of alcoholics, when they are young and when they are grown, suffer with many problems their counterparts in non-drinking families do not experience. For example, young children experience school problems, delinquency, fighting and difficulties developing relationships with peers (Booz-Allen and Hamilton Inc., 1974). Children who were stifled by hung-over or upset parents may develop a sense of shame or guilt about their feelings or their natural playfulness (Lawson, 1990). Some children also experience depression and suicidal tendencies. Others themselves become involved in alcohol and drug abuse (Booz-Allen and Hamilton Inc., 1974). Family members, hoping that the problem will disappear on its own, may ignore the substance abuse or speak of it in stilted or euphemistic terms. They fear that upsetting the abuser through confrontation may worsen the drinking or use of drugs. Some therapists and families report, 'It is as if an elephant is sitting in the living room and we are all too polite to mention the fact'. In the authors' experience, this behavior has been rigidly held to, even unto death of the patient.

> Juan Espinosa was astute at pointing out the relationship problems in his younger sister's family that led to her divorce. He described the pain that the divorce caused for the parents, children, and extended family. Somehow he remained blind to the pain that his drinking caused in his own family.
>
> In the very early stages of their marriage, Yolanda Espinosa minimized the effects of her husband's drinking on their family. She noticed her own increased irritation and anger at home, but she attributed her reactions to the stresses of rearing young children.

Poor and negative communication

Communication in the alcoholic family is often incongruent, unclear and negative in tone (Hecht, 1973; Jacob and Krahn, 1988). Depending on the personalities of family members and the length of time drinking has been a problem, different patterns of communication may evolve. For example, in the early stages of a family member's drinking, members may hesitate to confront the drinking or bring their reactions to the behavior out in the open. Later, family members may become angry and overtly hostile. After years of tolerating or trying to change the problem, family members may attempt to numb themselves to any feelings rather than risk experiencing the pain. Eventually, they may become cut-off or alienated from the substance abuser or from one another. The build-up of pain may become too great to experience; avoiding people who remind them of the painful situation may be the chosen way of escaping the worst.

> Mrs Espinosa spent many years trying to convince her husband he needed to stop drinking. She gave up, tried to numb herself to the pain of their negative interactions and focused on her life with her children. When drinking, Juan would sometimes become mean to her or the children. She reacted by keeping herself and her children at a safe distance from him as much as possible. This made him even angrier and intensified his meanness. Occasionally the children, distraught by their father's treatment, especially to their mother, would lash out in anger at their father.

Unbalanced roles

Family members of the abuser may fall into roles that are clearly defined and safe, but where animation, progression and adaptability are lacking. Several authors have described these roles (Black, 1981; Booz-Allen and Hamilton Inc., 1974; Wegscheider, 1981). One family member may act as the hero, accomplishing much, taking on many responsibilities and bringing glory to the family. Another member may become the placater or mascot who is intent on making others feel good. Another family member may play the role of scapegoat in order to take the focus off the alcoholic. The enabler hides the drinker's mistakes, promotes continued drinking or performs the duties of the drinker. The lost family member calls no attention to him or herself, merely receding into the background or getting involved with activities outside the family. These roles in families are not static, and family members may alternate or take on new roles (Jacob, 1992; Steinglass *et al.*, 1977), depending on factors such as the family member's changing stage of development, the nature of the current drinking patterns or changing family dynamics. Role labels may be helpful to the clinician to understand someone's behavior, to encourage a larger repertoire of behaviors or to inject humor as family members are playfully invited to look at their own actions. The labels should not be used, however, to narrowly define someone's personality (Rotunda *et al.*, 1995).

> Yolanda's life became totally focussed on her four children. She became father and mother to her children, attending parent-teacher conferences by herself, taking the children to church and practicing soccer or softball with them. She paid no attention to activities that used to be satisfying to her such as time with her girlfriends or the sewing she used to love. Juanita, the oldest daughter, was the family heroine, getting top grades in school and helping with her younger brother and sisters. When she turned 15, her role in the family changed. She began staying out late and smoking marijuana with her friends. Angel was the child whose problems with school performance distracted the parents from looking at their own relationship. There was always some new facet of Angel's problem to address. Cecilia had symptoms that surfaced occasionally, such as her nightmares. Maria tended to recede into the background, creating few waves and asking for little.

Rescuing, enabling and hiding the problem

Family members may rescue or make excuses for the substance abuser's behavior. In alcoholic families, loyalty to the drinker, fears for a provider's loss of employment, desires to cling to the illusion the drinking does not exist or hesitations to look at relationships may cause family members to hide the truth about their family member's drinking. At its most extreme, rescue may include keeping secret the illegal behaviors of the alcoholic or retrieving the abuser from jail. Rescued or saved from discovery, the drinker is allowed to continue, sometimes unnoticed by close contacts. For example, members may hide the true reasons for tardiness or absence of the drinker from work, thereby allowing the secret of the substance abuse to continue. Employers are familiar with the pattern of the spouse who calls in most Mondays to report a husband or wife who is 'ill' and unable to report for work. Parents may make excuses to children for abusing parents' non-participation in family activities. Members may even hide the seriousness of the problem from the drinker him or herself.

> In the case of Mrs Espinosa, she often picked her husband up from the floor after his collapse in a drunken stupor, and with her son's help carried him to bed. Her husband woke up not knowing what had happened the night before. For years she made excuses to his employers about why Juan was late or absent from work.

Angel would make excuses to his soccer coaches as to why his father, who had agreed to help out with the team, would not show up at practices. Juanita, embarrassed about her father's drinking, would not allow her friends to come visit her at her home.

Blaming

Family members often blame one another for the problems in the family. Users blame family members for creating problems or stresses that drive them to drink. Members may blame their substance-abusing family member for all the negative happenings in the family. Parents may blame children for acting-out in school or at home. Children may feel guilty because parents constantly fight about them. On the other hand, children may blame parents for lack of support or attention or the chaos at home. Researchers found that children have strong feelings of resentment and embarrassment because of their alcoholic parent and the instability in their familes (Booz-Allen and Hamilton Inc., 1974). The cycle of blame and bitterness is perpetuated.

Mrs Espinosa held many resentments against her husband. She resented his drinking and his inability to keep a job. She blamed him for their son Angel's symptoms of Attention Deficit-Hyperactivity Disorder (ADHD), their daughter Cecilia's nightmares and Maria's confusion about why her father was mean sometimes and other times very loving.

Enmeshment

Many families show patterns of enmeshment where members react automatically to other family members without planning their reactions, and believe they have some control over the others' behaviors. They imagine others think or act like they do. The drinking behavior interrupts normal family tasks, causes conflicts, shifts roles and requires adaptation to the drinking behaviors (Kaufman and Pattison, 1990). Additional symptoms of enmeshment are triangles and coalitions (Haley, 1977; Minuchin, 1974), where a child or other family member is brought into the conflict of the other two in a way that traps the child or family member in a loyalty conflict. Triangles and coalitions may shift depending on whether the alcoholic is actively drinking (Hudak et al., 1998).

In the Espinosa family, Yolanda turned to her son, Angel, and complained to him about his father, Juan. She incited Angel to anger at his father for not attending Angel's soccer games. Juan became angry toward his son for taking his mother's side and attended even fewer of his son's sporting events.

Alienation

Estrangement and even cut-off may result when family members become so angry towards one another that they decrease contact with or even refuse to be in the presence of the other family member. They build walls between themselves and other family members in order to protect themselves or loved ones from additional emotional or physical pain.

Juan and his older brother Ricardo grew up together and were buddies throughout childhood and adolescence, fishing together and playing soccer. In their adult years, Ricardo gave Juan lots of support, even lending him money when Juan lost his jobs. One time, Juan and his family moved in with Ricardo's family after Juan and Yolanda were evicted from their apartment. Juan never repaid the money he owed Ricardo, and when he asked Ricardo one more time for a loan, Ricardo exploded and refused to have any more contact with Juan. The fact that their father suffered from alcoholism most likely inflamed Ricardo's explosive response. The popular literature and newspaper advice columns such as 'Dear Abby' are replete with examples of family members who refuse to speak over years if not decades related to substance-abusing behavior.

Depression and stress

Symptoms of depression and stress take their toll on the entire family of the alcoholic (Kaufman and Pattison, 1990). Substance abusers sometimes become depressed in response to increased alienation by family members or the guilt they feel for continued drinking. Their depression may lead to more drinking in order to ameliorate the pain of the guilt or estrangement. When Ricardo asked Juan and his family to leave his home, Juan fell into a deep depression, feeling rejected by the brother who had always been his advocate. Alcohol, of course, is a depressant itself. A common dilemma in treatment is the chicken/egg: 'Did they drink because of depression or are they depressed because of drinking?' The usual recommendation is to 'dry before you try ... antidepressants'. Family members, too, may experience symptoms of depression and stress. Some may even experience suicidal tendencies or actually attempt suicide.

The Espinosas' daughter, Cecilia, began having nightmares after the dismissal from her uncle's home, and Mrs Espinosa's headaches worsened. Eleven-year-old Angel Espinosa's school performance declined from previous functioning. He was brought to his primary care provider for evaluation for ADHD. His teacher noted that he was not concentrating on his schoolwork and was very easily distracted. Although he was new to the school, a factor that could explain his behavior, reports from his previous school did not indicate problems with concentration. Angel's attitude was not a problem; he did not seem to intentionally ignore his assignments. The primary care provider discovered that Angel's problem in school worsened as his father increased his level of drinking and decreased his time with Angel and the family.

Some family members respond to their depressed feelings by drinking to alleviate the pain of the depression. In the Espinosa family, Juan's mother was depressed. Mrs Espinosa often wondered if Juan drank to alleviate the pain he felt in reaction to his mother's depression.

Acting-out

Children and spouses of alcoholics often drift into self-defeating, destructive, or rebellious behaviors. Subconsciously, family members may want to defy the alcoholic, challenge them to pay attention or escalate the family problems to the point that finally outside help is sought.

Fifteen-year-old Juanita Espinosa began staying out until early morning hours with her friends. One time when she came home, her mother detected on her the smell of marijuana. Juanita denied using marijuana, saying her friends had been smoking but she had not. In the case of Mrs Espinosa, she also encountered a period where she went through a stage of 'acting-out'. Before her father died and while he was ill, Yolanda became very depressed. She was also very angry toward Juan during this time for not participating in their family life. For two months, she drank to alleviate her pain and suffering. Fortunately, she awoke to the fact that she was destroying herself and hurting her family and she quit drinking.

Punishing behaviors

Families find many ways to punish their alcoholic members for their drinking. Some families plan social events at times the drinker will be unavailable. Other families withhold family resources such as time, money, tools or emotional support that they would otherwise share with the alcoholic. Couples' usual sexual relationships may disappear as the spouses of the alcoholics become dejected and angry. Families may become so resentful of the alcoholic that they even exclude the drinker from family inheritances.

> Juan Espinosa's brother, Ricardo, was so angry at Juan about his drinking when they lived together that Ricardo destroyed all of the beer Juan had hidden in his basement. Mrs Espinosa, frustrated and tired of her lonely role in the family, had no interest in a sexual relationship with her husband. She had no desire to give him what he seemed to want most from her.

Lifecycle stagnation

Families naturally change over time. They adjust to the births and deaths of family members, to the challenges of caring for members who become dependent and to managing economic burdens of the family. At different stages of the family lifecycle, new challenges come into play. Clinicians who understand the normal phases of the family will be able to assess whether the family in treatment is adjusting well to transitions. Alcoholic families face special challenges as they adjust to new lifecycle stages while there is active drinking or dysfunctional behavior on the part of family members.

Tracking typical family development is worthwhile in the same way that tracking an infant's growth and development is useful – clinicians will know if the family is adapting well, or if interventions are warranted. Examples are described from the stages of the newly-formed couple, the family with young children, and the family with adolescents. The newly-formed couple face the practical challenges of getting along at home and becoming economic partners. The emotional and relational challenges they face are to build a commitment to one another and shift allegiances from their families of origin to their newly-formed family. Crises that may take place at this juncture are conflicts with in-laws (Gerson, 1995). At the next stage, the family with young children, the practical challenges faced are organizing the household for rearing children and managing financial obligations. The emotional and relational challenges are accepting the new family members, maintaining the marital unit while taking on parental responsibilities and integrating grandparents into the family configuration (Gerson, 1995). At the stage of the family with adolescents, the members need to face the challenge of the adolescent's unavailability and less predictable routines. The emotional and relational challenges are to maintain contact with the adolescent while encouraging more independence. A possible crisis at this time is that of adolescent rebellion.

As Brown and Weston (1995) have noted, the impact of a major illness such as substance abuse on the family will vary according to where they find themselves in the family lifecycle. When faced with developmental challenges at different stages, members in alcoholic families may resist or fail to accomplish these challenges because of fear that family life may worsen or because there is an absence of resources to meet the challenges. Customary family, community and work supports may have disappeared in the alcoholic family. Depending on the seriousness of the drinking problem and the length of time of the abuse, the family's energy for responding to lifecycle challenges may wither. In the early stages of a member's drinking, there may be marital strain while in the chronic phase of the drinking, there may be anger and outright hostility in the married couple (Krestan and Bepko, 1989) and the extended family. Likewise, in chronic phases of the problem there may be a decreased chance of attaining intimacy in a partnership, an important quality of successful married life. In the chronic phases, parenting responsibilities of the abuser may suffer and, by default, the spouse of the drinker becomes responsible for all parental tasks. Children may, in essence, lose their parent. Likewise, adults who are drinking may abandon the mission of caring for their aging parents if they are preoccupied with drinking. Family members who take on the drinker's lifecycle responsibilities, such as the spouses who care for their in-laws, may be faced with neglecting their own development, such as progression in their careers.

The Espinosa family is at the lifecycle stages of the family with young children and the family with adolescents. In their family sessions after referral for counseling, Mrs Espinosa acknowledged that she was clinging to her children at a time when they needed more encouragement toward independence. She was still grieving for the loss of her father since his death nine months before. In their new town, she had no friends. As Juan's drinking worsened, Yolanda felt more lonely and isolated. Practically the only time she felt truly alive was when she was with her children. Angel was on the soccer team, but she often felt like he was 'needed at home'. Angel sometimes felt that he needed to stay home from his activities to 'protect' his mother from his father's meanness. In essence, the lifecycle challenges of children maintaining contact with parents while encouraging children's independence were not met.

Violence and abuse

Taboos and inhibitions usually keep us from hurting each other through violence, aggression, sexual abuse or physical abuse. In the drinker, these taboos and inhibitions may be drowned in alcohol. Parents may seek physical contact with the child in inappropriate ways, for example, in order to gratify their own needs for closeness (Booz-Allen and Hamilton Inc., 1974). Alcohol quashes skills and reasoning capabilities ordinarily used in solving relationship problems. Dysfunctional family dynamics, such as ignoring the problem, enmeshment and alienation, lead to the escalation of anger and intimidation.

When Mrs Espinosa's primary care practitioner asked her to comment on incidences of violence or abuse in the family, Yolanda tearfully described a time when her husband was about to drive their 15-year-old daughter, Juanita, to her school softball game to watch her play. Juan was drunk and Mrs Espinosa refused to give him the keys to the car. Juan shoved her. Juanita, afraid for her mother's safety, grabbed her softball bat and wrestled her father to the floor, keeping the bat to Juan's back. Juanita held her father in this position for some time until he began to become sober again. Primary care practitioners need to regularly assess for violence in the family (Leonard and Jacob, 1988; O'Farrell, 1993).

Family dissolution

The instability, alienation and lack of intimacy or purpose in alcoholic families may lead, finally, to the break-up of the family. Alcoholic members sometimes abandon the family due to shame or guilt, or to be free to drink unobserved. Nondrinking spouses may become completely disillusioned by the continued drinking, and lose hope for improvement in their relationships. As children leave to escape the drinking, there may be little reason for the family to stay together.

Mrs Espinosa admitted in counseling she had packed her bags on many occasions, but always came back. Recently, she had again been debating with herself the merits of moving out with her children. Even with the family in counseling and Juan in recovery, Mrs Espinosa was unsure about the longevity of her marriage.

Resilience

Many alcoholic families show surprising resilience at points in their development. Some families, for example, are able to go about the tasks of rearing children even when alcohol is a problem in the family. Some children show success in school and in their social relationships despite difficulties at home. Children's successes are often attributed to supportive family members other than the alcoholics (Booz-Allen and Hamilton Inc., 1974; Simmons, 1991) or to mentors for the children (O'Sullivan, 1991). Family researchers interviewed adolescents who overcame dire circumstances in their families, including alcoholism and drug abuse. They identified seven ways adolescents showed resilience: insight, independence, initiative, relating to healthy individuals, creativity, humor and morality (Jacobs and Wolin, 1991; Wolin and Wolin, 1993). Some children of alcoholics describe becoming independent at an early age and maturing more quickly than their friends (Booz-Allen and Hamilton Inc., 1974).

Many of these aspects of resilience were found in the Espinosa children. They showed amazing initiative and independence – they were always at school on time, did their homework most of the time and took part in school and extracurricular activities. In addition, they sought out relationships with healthy individuals. The two older children established good relationships with their male coaches who became mentors for them. The two younger children asked regularly to spend time with their Uncle Ricardo and his family; there they were consistently loved and supported. Adults in dysfunctional situations may show resilience as well. Yolanda and Juan had creative and humorous sides that emerged in their singing and dancing. The two had met on the dance floor when they were in their twenties. Even at the worst of times in their family life, they periodically put aside their resentments and the whole family danced to Mexican salsa music. The strong moral values Yolanda and Juan inherited from their families of origin, such as concern for others, remained important to them personally and were a legacy they intended to pass on to their children.

Families are more likely to show resilience if they engage in regular family rituals. Rituals, such as routine daily activities including mealtimes, holiday celebrations, birthdays, anniversaries and reunions, bring family members together and provide a structure to family life. Through rituals, family members' feelings of alienation decrease and their sense of family identity increases (Imber-Black *et al.*, 1988; Rotunda *et al.*, 1995; Wolin *et al.*, 1980). Researchers investigating families where one parent was an alcoholic found that those families who preserved family rituals did not transmit alcoholism to their offspring (Wolin *et al.*, 1979). An important factor when encouraging family rituals is for those family events not to be centered around alcohol.

Genetics

The last decade has seen an explosion of research in the genetics of alcoholism. An excellent summary of this research can be found in Chapter 2. Schuckit's research (1999) indicates that first-degree relatives of alcoholics have a three- to four-fold increase in the risk of alcoholism. Still, it must be noted that roughly half of the risk of alcoholism is related to culture, family influence and environment. In regards to family influences, many is the time that each of the authors has heard the desperate plea, 'I swore that I would never drink and end up like my father!' from someone who is being detoxed from doing just that. In any family treatment it is important to reinforce the increased risk of alcohol abuse by children of substance-abusing parents. Often the rejoinder is: 'Doc, it'll never happen to me!'

Assessing the family

Healthcare providers need to be attuned to stress-related illnesses and problems in family members of substance abusers. Many symptoms may signal problems. Vague somatic complaints such as aches and pains are typical. Changes in family members' school or work performance may signify change in the substance abusers' habits or family dynamics that have changed. Children may not reach developmental milestones as predicted or regress to earlier levels of behavior. The child with secondary enuresis is an example of regression back to an earlier stage of development. Adolescents may either act-out, such as with drugs or sexual promiscuity, or they may become reclusive or depressed. The spouse of the alcoholic may be at risk from substance abuse or ignoring self-care, resulting in problems such as obesity or illness. The earliest problems associated with alcohol abuse are often relationship and work difficulties (Steinglass *et al.*, 1987). The practitioner should be alert to consideration of substance abuse when problems such as major difficulties with bosses, marital disputes or parent–child conflicts become apparent.

To stay abreast of these family and medical issues, the healthcare providers will need to routinely ask about how things are going in the family. Families are usually the first to recognize substance abuse problems, and practitioners should routinely ask members if anyone in their family is drinking or using drugs. At regular intervals, the practitioner may want to have family conferences so as to have a full view of the family and medical issues. Family assessment tools such as the genogram (McGoldrick *et al.*, 1999) can be invaluable for tracking family dynamics, health status and lifecycle stages of the various family members. Collecting genogram information across at least three generations will reveal much about the family system. It is important, however, to remember that many patients and families do not think to include alcoholism or other substance abuse as a family disease, and the interviewer must ask specifically whether anyone in the family is a heavy drinker or uses drugs. When the Espinosa family was interviewed using the genogram, it was discovered that

Juan was not the only drinker in the family. His father and father-in-law were both heavy drinkers as well (*see* Figure 5.1). One or several family members may be interviewed to provide this information. A brief genogram interview includes the presenting problem, living arrangements of the family, family history, major life events, family relationships (e.g. cut-offs, alliances, dominance/submission patterns, marital patterns, parent–child patterns), family roles, family strengths and questions about individual functioning. Details of interview approaches and interpretation are found in McGoldrick *et al.* (1999).

Family reactions to the drinking are important to assess. Questions such as 'How much pain has been caused by the drinking?' (Hudak *et al.*, 1998), and 'Who is most affected by the drinking?' will reveal much about the family's reactions. The answers may signal the family members' readiness to address the problem of addiction and may energize the practitioner toward investing time in plans for intervention.

Dysfunction in the workplace

Maladaptive behaviors often carry over into the workplace as well. Shortly after the formation of AA in the mid 1930s came the development of Occupational Alcoholism (OA), which drew AA into the workplace in the 1940s. These programs developed into what are now termed Employee Assistance Programs (EAPs). With her request for counseling, Mrs Espinosa took a step in the direction of healing. EAPs are not only for substance abuse but any issue, marital, psychological or even financial, that may be impacting the individual's productivity. EAPs provide brief, several-session screening, counseling and/or referral. Substance-abusing employees are often loners trying to hide their problem. They are often less productive and less involved in the company and interact less with other employees.

Carl Etheridge was Juan Espinosa's immediate supervisor at the plant. He thought he had noted the smell of alcohol and, at times, marijuana on Juan. But Juan had managed to artfully deflect all of his supervisor's careful inquiries. After all, the competition was between a seasoned veteran with years of experience, Juan, and Carl with a few hours of supervisory training. Carl felt a grim sort of satisfaction when an injury led to Juan's discovery. With Carl's help, the Medical Review Officer was able to direct the Espinosas to his company's EAP, and counseling began. A few days after Juan's discovery, Carl received a call from Eric Danforth, the company's EAP counselor. Eric explained that for Juan to eventually recover and return to the workforce, Carl needed to be a willing partner in Juan's recovery. This would, Eric warned, require some additional time for education for Carl. After a few moments of hesitation, but mindful of the labor short-age of skilled workers, Carl agreed.

A few weeks later, Eric Danforth appeared at the factory with Juan in tow. But what a difference in Juan, Carl noted. The old Juan was often sullen, pale and withdrawn. This Juan was sporting a smile, albeit a little sheepish, making eye contact and looking better than Carl would have believed possible.

Securing a place in Carl's office overlooking the shop floor, Carl had one more surprise – Juan began by apologizing for the trouble he caused. Embarrassed, Carl tried to wave it away. 'No', Juan persisted, 'It's part of the treatment to apologize to those I've harmed.' Then he finished. There was a moment's awkward pause. Carl tried to fill it by asking about what Juan has been doing. Juan nodded to Eric.

'Juan has been in intensive day treatment for the last month,' Eric began. 'This included one-on-one counseling, group counseling, exercise and daily attendance at AA meetings. He will be ready to return to work next week, but as a condition of employment, he'll be subject to random drug and alco-hol testing. We'll supervise that from the EAP office but if you have reason to be concerned, you can call us and we'll arrange one for you.'

Carl tried to object. 'Eric, Juan managed to dodge me the whole ten months he was here. How am I supposed to diagnose a slip?'

Eric smiled. 'Well first, I hope you're a lot more suspicious now.' Carl nodded. 'There is a long and formal definition for alcoholism and substance abuse with various criteria, but I can boil it down to what I tell other people who flunk their drug test. If your use is interfering with your life and other activities, you've got a problem. Then I point out that they may lose their job over the failed test and *that* is definitely a problem.'

'Amen!' Juan jumped in.

Eric continued, 'You may recall that I had called a few weeks ago and asked for Juan's time and attendance and disciplinary records, Carl?' Carl nodded. Eric pulled out a sheaf of papers as he continued. 'I also cross-refer-enced Juan's medical claims from personnel and I thought you might be interested in the results. I do have Juan's and his wife's permission to do this, right Juan?' Juan nodded.

'First, you'll note that this is not Juan's first accident. Actually, it is his third.' Eric glanced at a report and smiled ruefully. 'In this one I see that Juan bumped someone with a forklift and *he* was the one who got drug tested. The interesting thing, however, is how common this is. Substance-abusing employees are much more likely to have accidents in the workplace. Actually, they are about three and a half times more likely to have an acci-dent than non-abusing employees (Berenstein and Mahoney, 1989). They also have absenteeism rates as much as two to eight times the sober em-ployee (Berenstein and Mahoney, 1989; Floren, 1994).

'That is why our State adopted a drug-free workplace act. The employer gets a discount on Worker's Compensation insurance. The law also shifts the burden of proof to the employee. This means that the assumption was that if the employee is at work, the law assumes the business is at fault. If the employee, Juan here, for example, fails the drug test, he has to prove that he didn't cause the accident.' Eric smiled sarcastically. 'I'm not a lawyer, I never played one on TV, but I'm told that is a tough legal standard to prove.'

Eric shuffled his papers and pulled out some medical claims. He spread them out in front of Carl. 'Work is not the only place where there is a problem. Look here at the medical claims. Juan was in the hospital twice: once for a bleeding ulcer and another for a motorcycle wreck. You'll notice he was legally intoxicated in the emergency department after the wreck.' Eric looked over the sheets and sighed. He held up a hospital discharge sheet. 'You'll notice that in neither case at discharge is alcoholism listed as a diagnosis. The average patient sees over three doctors before one will diagnose alcoholism. In addition, doctors are often afraid to list the diagnosis for fear of not getting paid or stigmatizing the patient. You know that we now have laws that require equal funding for both medical and psychiatric treatment, but they still exclude substance abuse. That is sort of silly, really, when you consider that substance-abusing patients consume about eight times the medical resources of non-abusing patients. Yet another cost to your company. Overall, substance abuse, counting drug tests, lost productivity and medical claims, is estimated to cost American business hundreds of billions of dollars. Alcohol-related deaths alone cost $75 billion and the cost to the alcoholic is a loss of nine to 22 years of life' (Fleming *et al.*, 1997).

'Jeez, Eric,' Carl expostulated, 'I never knew. Why don't companies do better on this sort of thing?'

'Well, they are. The whole EAP movement grew out of several companies back in the forties who adapted AA to Industry, calling it OA for Occupational Alcoholism. Now we do short-term counseling for almost anything from substance abuse to marital problems to financial counseling, and it is usually free to you and your family. But, to answer your question, companies are often like families. The same dynamics apply. They can be in denial, or be over-involved and enable the abuser to continue their downward spiral. Usually, however, the workplace is the last place that the employees will allow their chemical dependency to show, since it is how they pay for their supply. But, like Juan's case, the employer has the best 'hook' for the same reason. Employers can pressure employees to return or face job loss. Employers are often invited to be part of an intervention if possible because they carry such a big stick. Of course, employees have a 'hook' too, in that if employees return to work, companies save in recruiting and retraining costs.'

Eric gathered up his papers as he continued. 'Part of Juan's recovery process will be that he will be required by my office to attend 90 AA meetings over the next 90 days. I note that your work shifts are 10 hours long. I'd like to ask that you accommodate Juan under the Americans with Disabilities Act (ADA) to let him off an hour early to connect with his AA group. When he finishes the 90 days, he can go on his day off.'

Carl shrugged, 'Nine tenths of Juan is better than no Juan. But' he continued, 'am I going to have to treat Juan as a disabled person from now on? I can't have him pulling this stuff in the future. Can I, Juan?' Juan shook his head vigorously.

'No,' Eric noted. 'Drug testing is specifically excluded from the ADA. Likewise, if you have a drug and alcohol policy forbidding alcohol while working, it'd apply to Juan like anyone else. And, of course, these last few weeks Juan has been taking advantage of yet another workplace law, the Family Medical Leave Act, because he used up all his sick time in those other cases. Well, that about wraps us up. Any questions for either of you?'

Juan jumped to his feet, extending his hand to Carl. Flashing a smile, he said, 'Many thanks for the second chance.' He shook hands with Eric and quickly left, closing the door behind him. Eric looked after him, musing.

'You know, it's funny how different cultures deal with this. Some Hispanics like Juan grow up with alcohol. Theirs is a Catholic culture that doesn't see alcohol as a forbidden substance like us Protestants that settled this area. For them, alcohol is part of life, well, at least for men, since it is mostly the men who drink. To them it is a matter of *machismo*, sometimes even cultural pride. It is a tough thing, almost unmanly, for them to make the first admission of AA, "that we are powerless over alcohol". Likewise they are family-oriented and protective. To admit that they were themselves the cause of harm and apologize is particularly tough. And finding a counselor who understands addictive disease *and* is sensitive to their culture in this region is about impossible. Thank goodness, it looks like things are working out for Juan. I think he's off to a really good start.'

Conclusion

Sir William Osler once stated that, 'It is more important what patient has the disease than what disease the patient has' (Porter, 1997). In recent years, patient-centered medicine has focused our attention on understanding the whole patient, and not just disease pathology. Increasing numbers of primary care providers, family counselors and employee assistance counselors are working to understand disease in the context of the patient and the patient in the context of the family, society and environment.

All parts of the family-work-provider system are touched by the problems of alcohol. Many providers, using a strictly medical/rational model, have been frustrated to the point of cynicism in dealing with chemically dependent patients. We hope that we have provided a rationale for demonstrating the value of the patient-centered model in dealing with patients with substance abuse disorders. Incorporating this broader approach will lead healthcare providers to collaborate with the patients and families in a spirit of empathy, compassion and mutual respect. Addressing multiple elements of the systems in which our patients function will be essential in intervening successfully with substance abuse problems and preventing problems from being transmitted to the next generations. In our experience, there are few more grateful patients than those families who manage, with the help of caring professionals, to transcend the disease of chemical addiction.

6

Health promotion and prevention of substance abuse

J Paul Seale

Editor's introduction

We now turn our attention to the fourth component of patient-centered medicine: health promotion and disease prevention as they relate to substance abuse. Health promotion refers to the way in which the patient-centered clinician looks for ways to increase the level of good health, vitality and resilience of persons without substance abuse problems or predisposing risk factors. Disease prevention, as defined by McWilliam and Freeman (1995), encompasses three aspects: risk avoidance for those who are currently low-risk users; risk reduction for those in the at-risk category; and early identification of those with early substance disorders. In this chapter, we will examine how emerging findings in substance abuse prevention and advances in the development of effective screening instruments can be used by the patient-centered clinician to maximize the impact of this key element of the clinical method.

The need for health promotion

Substance abuse is a systems problem which involves individuals, their genetic risk, their individual vulnerability due to life stage and personal stressors; interpersonal relationships within and outside the family and environmental influences which encourage or discourage substance use (Berenson, 1976; Steinglass *et al.*, 1987). This system has its own stability and equilibrium, with the substance abuse disorder impacting not only the health of the individual, but also reverberating through all aspects of the patient's life, including the family, the work setting and at times the larger community. The healthcare provider, as a part of this system, has the potential of touching the patient in health-promoting ways so that the patient's health behaviors and other elements of this system shift in a positive direction.

The patient-oriented clinician must approach prevention efforts with an understanding of the whole person in context (Weston *et al.*, 1989), being sensitive to important factors in the patient's life which determine the response to health promotion messages. For example, the clinician must clarify the patient's perception of their health status. Research has demonstrated a strong positive correlation between self-reported perceived health status and a health-promoting lifestyle (Gillis, 1993). Equally important is the patient's perception of the extent to which he or she is responsible for and in control of his or her own health and able to make changes that will improve health status (McWilliam and Freeman, 1995). These two factors have been found to be the most powerful predictors of a health-promoting lifestyle (Gillis, 1993), and facilitate the clinician's attempts to function as a facilitator and educator in the process of health promotion.

The patient-centered physician must avoid the temptation to develop standardized lectures which are applied to all patients regarding their risk of substance use disorders. It is crucial to use the patient's world as the starting point, including their individual risk profile, their beliefs in relation to health and illness, the value placed on health (Calnan, 1988) and the role which alcohol or drugs play in the individual's life. Perceived benefits of the use of alcohol and drugs, for example as a means of recreation or stress management, must be weighed against potential harm to health, family and job performance. Barriers to achieving a health-promoting lifestyle, such as the difficulty of achieving abstinence or the potential impact of abstinence on relationships with others who use alcohol and drugs, must be recognized and dealt with. Individuals who use alcohol or drugs are often surrounded by friends and family who also use or abuse psychoactive substances, and may benefit from considering the possible reactions of others around them should they decide to alter their substance use, and how to respond to such reactions.

This chapter will examine recent findings from the field of substance abuse prevention and seek to elucidate how the patient-centered method can enhance the application of these findings to day-to-day clinical practice.

Health promotion and risk avoidance activities with teens and pre-teens

The primary care practitioner should be an active agent in health promotion activities in both the clinical setting and the community (Jernigan, 1991; Jernigan *et al.*, 1989). There is now compelling evidence that the younger individuals are when they begin to drink, the higher their risk of alcohol abuse and alcoholism (Grant, 1997a). Therefore, interventions which delay the onset of drinking can have significant long-term impact. In order to intervene in a patient-centered manner, however, the clinician must start by identifying the patient's own beliefs regarding alcohol and drug use by asking questions such as: Do you think using drugs is dangerous to your health? What about alcohol? Have you ever tried alcohol or marijuana? If so, what was it like? Do you have any religious or spiritual beliefs that influence your desire to use or not use alcohol or drugs? Do you have any friends or family who have had problems related to alcohol or drug use? By obtaining this kind of information, the clinician can tailor health promotion messages to the patient's individual context. The following list provides a menu of health promotion interventions that practitioners might wish to utilize as a part of their day-to-day clinical activities.

- Provide factual information about substance abuse disorders to adolescents, pre-adolescents and their parents as a routine part of patient education activities, especially in younger patients who often present with relatively minor, acute illnesses. Brief visits for physical examinations for school, sports involvement or summer camp provide ideal opportunities for such activities. Patient education materials can be made available to patients both in the waiting-room and the examination room (Jernigan *et al.*, 1989), and should target both parents and younger patients. Quality patient education materials can be obtained from sources such as the National Council on Alcoholism (NCA), and should be reinforced with verbal messages from the practitioner. Providing young people with accurate information can have a powerful effect in changing their drinking behavior, as demonstrated by studies which show that the correction of exaggerated misperceptions of others' drinking behavior can significantly reduce binge drinking and its consequences among college students (Agnostinelli *et al.*, 1995; Haines and Spear, 1996; Steffian, 1999). Important facts to reinforce include the following:

  - alcohol and drug use carry significant health risks, and are highly associated with accidents, injuries and unprotected sex in adolescence and young adulthood
  - delaying the onset of drinking, smoking and drug use significantly reduces the risk of development of alcohol and drug abuse
  - association with peers who do not drink, smoke or use other drugs decreases the risk that adolescents will begin to drink, smoke or use
  - while it may appear that many students drink large amounts on a regular basis, research indicates that most students, even at the college level, do not drink at all or drink only one or two days per week, and drink four drinks or less when they do drink (Perkins *et al.*, 1999; Steffian 1999).

- Inform patients of the benefits of avoiding alcohol, tobacco and drug use during the adolescent period. Adolescents are more likely to respond to education which emphasizes short-term benefits, such as decreasing their risk of accidents, sexually transmitted diseases or unwanted pregnancy, rather than long-term health consequences such as preventing cirrhosis or alcohol-related cancers. In countries such as the US, where alcohol use is illegal before age 21, the patient has the added advantage of avoiding problems with legal authorities by observing such a policy.

- Encourage teens and pre-teens to plan and participate in alcohol-free recreational activities such as athletics, movies, dances, ski trips, roller skating, bowling and beach parties. Formal prevention studies have demonstrated that youth who are involved in planning and implementing alcohol-free activities are significantly less likely to use alcohol than their peers (Komro *et al.*, 1996).

- Encourage involvement in religious activities and personal spiritual development. Spirituality has been described as a missing component in many substance abuse-prevention programs (Henson, 1998), while religious beliefs have been clearly demonstrated to be a significant factor in determining alcohol and drug use in cultures around the world. In the US, personal religiosity and involvement in church activities have been found to significantly decrease the risk of adolescent substance use (Cochran, 1992; Cochran and Akers, 1989; Jessor, 1983; Kutter and McDermott, 1997). In Israel, Moslem and Druze youth who do not drink report that the religious injunction of their faith and perceived harmful health consequences are the most important reasons for abstinence (Moore and Weiss, 1995). Religious activities for youth now include not only church participation but also religious coffee houses, home-study groups, campus clubs, and contemporary religious music and concerts. The patient-centered clinician should feel free to ask patients about their personal beliefs and religious tradition, while always demonstrating respect for the individual's convictions. Those interested in spiritual matters should be encouraged to develop their personal spirituality by involvement in formal and informal religious activities such as church, Bible studies and religious clubs.

- Encourage positive interactions between parents and adolescents, as well as the development of family norms or policies regarding use of alcohol, tobacco and other drugs. Family factors that appear to have protective effects against alcohol problems include high levels of parental support and monitoring, positive adolescent–parent communication and active parental nurturance of teenage children (Barnes *et al.*, 1995). Studies also indicate that teens whose parents establish and communicate norms which discourage alcohol and tobacco use are less likely to drink and smoke (Peterson *et al.*, 1995). The clinician may assist interested parents and teens by providing examples of policies or formal contracts which other families have found useful.

- Utilize role-play techniques to help interested teens and pre-teens develop resistance skills. The clinician should establish a dialogue with patients about situations where friends or classmates have tried to pressure them into drinking or using drugs, or situations where this might occur in the future. They can then work together with the patient to develop a series of responses they might use in such situations, and even role-play such a situation to allow them to practice their responses. This kind of skills training in resistance skills has been shown to result in significant reductions in adolescent drinking (Graham *et al.*, 1990; Hansen *et al.*, 1988).
- Encourage the use of safe-drinking limits among those patients who decide to drink alcohol. As noted in Chapter 1, limits currently recommended by the NIAAA are as follows: for men, no more than 14 total drinks per week and no more than four drinks per occasion; for women, no more than seven drinks per week and no more than three drinks per occasion (NIAAA, 1995). Special emphasis should be given to avoiding drinking in high-risk situations, such as while operating motor vehicles. Alcohol-related motor vehicle accidents are one of the leading causes of death and injury in teens and young adults (Hingson and Howland, 1989; Williams and Lillis, 1988).

Identifying at-risk adolescents and pre-teenagers

While it is now clear that genetic factors play a key role in the risk of this disorder, many other variables also influence individuals' psychoactive chemical use patterns and whether or not they become abusive. For example, genetically predisposed individuals who never use mood-altering substances such as alcohol, tobacco or marijuana will never develop substance abuse disorders. For this reason, the prevalence of substance abuse problems is markedly lower in countries where religious and cultural norms strongly discourage alcohol and drug use, and among women in cultures where it is culturally unacceptable for women to drink to the point of intoxication.

It is not necessarily the presence or absence of one or a combination of risk factors in an individual, but rather their interaction with each other, in combination with the individual's setting and developmental stage, that results in problems related to chemical use in a given individual (Zucker, 1994). One of the challenges facing the individual practitioner is to step back and attempt to view as many aspects of the individual patient's system as possible when assessing risk and attempting preventive interventions. The following is a list of risk factors which have been demonstrated to increase patients' risk of developing substance abuse disorders.

- **Genetically-determined individual differences.** As highlighted in Chapter 2, individuals with a family history of substance abuse are at higher risk of developing substance abuse disorders than the general population. Individuals with this risk factor can easily be identified by including questions about alcohol and drug disorders in the routine family history and genogram. The high prevalence and serious impact of substance abuse justify including it in the list of disorders routinely screened for in the family history, such as hypertension, heart disease, cancer and diabetes. Practitioners should be careful in the way questions regarding alcohol and drug problems are phrased. The question, 'Are there any heavy drinkers, alcohol or drug problems in your family?' is much more likely to gather the desired information than use of such stigmatized terms as alcoholism or drug addiction.

- **Other individual differences.** Other individual characteristics which are not necessarily genetically determined may also contribute to the development of a substance abuse disorder. These characteristics include a predisposition to negative moods, a tendency toward sensation seeking, impulsivity, impaired coping skills and the expectancy of reinforcement from alcohol. Adolescents with decreased self-esteem, those who have experienced school failure and those manifesting socially deviant behaviors are also at higher risk of developing substance abuse disorders (Sher, 1994).

- **Family influences.** Family factors that have been found to predict substance use and abuse during adolescence include parental alcohol consumption, poor family management practices, parental attitudes and norms which are favorable towards adolescent alcohol and tobacco use, the involvement of children in parental alcohol use, family disruption, relationship problems between the parents, lack of parental support of children and inability of parents to facilitate socialization and the development of the children's values (Newcomb, 1994; Peterson *et al.*, 1995).

- **Peer influences.** The increasing importance of peer relationships is a normal part of adolescent development. Peers can have either a positive or negative impact on the development of substance abuse problems. Many adolescents tend to look to their peers rather than to their parents for help and advice in important life decisions, and their perceptions about the acceptability of alcohol use are heavily influenced by the attitudes of those peers. Alcohol and drug use have been correlated with association with peers who use alcohol; peer pressure to drink, smoke or use drugs; peer rejection and involvement in deviant peer groups (Barnes *et al.*, 1995; Jacob and Leonard, 1994; Klitzner *et al.*, 1988; Marks *et al.*, 1992). As noted above, even erroneous perceptions of peers' drinking behavior appear to affect alcohol consumption among adolescents. Surveys not only confirm that college students tend to overestimate the prevalence of heavy drinking among their peers, but also show an association between exaggerated perceptions of the norm and greater personal alcohol abuse (Perkins and Wechsler, 1996).

- **Cultural and societal influences.** Adolescent alcohol and drug use is highly influenced by a number of cultural and societal influences which may encourage psychoactive substance use. In many segments of Western society, the decision to use alcohol and learning how to drink are perceived as a rite of passage into adulthood (Howard *et al.*,1995), with regular alcohol consumption at social functions beginning during the mid to late teens.

Risk reduction interventions for high-risk youth

The presence of any of the risk factors noted does not obviate the need for implementing the health promotion steps listed above. If anything, these interventions become even more important in the at-risk youth. High-risk youth need accurate information about substance abuse disorders, especially their own genetic predisposition to develop these disorders. The benefits of avoiding alcohol and drugs, especially during adolescence, are even greater in their case. They should be strongly encouraged to plan and participate in alcohol-free recreational activities. At this point, challenges may emerge, especially for those who are already beginning to center their recreational activities around alcohol or drugs. The clinician may need to establish a dialogue with them about the particular risks of their own alcohol or drug use, and to brainstorm about alternative recreational activities that would be of interest to them. Involvement in religious activities and development of their own spirituality may be either preventive or therapeutic, if they are beginning to develop problems related to their substance use. Religious-based programs such as Teen Challenge and the Palmer Drug Abuse Program have been effective treatment interventions for thousands of substance-abusing youth. Family-based interventions may be a major challenge if parents are themselves abusing alcohol or drugs. Research on resilient youth has indicated, however, that many resilient youth may avoid problems with alcohol or drugs by identifying healthy adult role models outside their nuclear family. Role-playing resistance skills may be important in a different context, such as resisting the temptation to experiment with more dangerous substances. The clinician may wish to challenge at-risk youth to seek out or spend more time with non-using friends, and to brainstorm about how to explain to substance-abusing friends who ask why they do not come around any more. For at-risk youth who choose to drink, the clinician may wish not only to encourage safe drinking limits but also a periodic screening visit to assess whether alcohol-related problems are emerging. Finally, the practitioner may wish to implement more intensive psychosocial interventions designed to increase self-esteem, assist in coping with negative emotions, improve school performance and social skills, modify expectancies about alcohol and other drug use and address early anti-social behavior. It may often be appropriate to involve other members of the healthcare team such as social workers, psychologists and educational specialists to address individual needs which lie beyond the expertise of the practitioner.

Screening for substance abuse disorders

In addition to adopting a pro-active position in regard to health promotion and risk reduction, primary care providers must be prepared to screen their patients for substance abuse problems. While patients with many other disorders present seeking diagnosis and treatment, substance-abusing patients are often in denial, not consciously aware that a problem exists, or even consciously working to thwart a diagnosis. Patients with drug and alcohol problems are twice as likely to consult a primary care physician compared to patients without such problems (Rush, 1989). Universal screening for substance abuse problems, especially alcohol abuse, is now being promoted in all primary care settings (NIAAA, 1995; Parish, 1997). This may be done as a part of the clinical interview, or by use of simple written questionnaires. For example, the Health Screening Survey (HSS) (Fleming and Barry, 1991) is a 17-question instrument which assesses alcohol use patterns and consequences but which also includes parallel questions regarding exercise, tobacco use and efforts at weight control. The use of appropriate screening questions assists the clinician in determining whether the patient is a low-risk user, at-risk user, problem user or is chemically dependent, as outlined in Figure 1.1, Chapter 1. This determination then allows the clinician to decide whether the appropriate intervention is health promotion, risk reduction, or treatment intervention.

Crucial information to be obtained during the screening interview includes whether patients use alcohol, tobacco or drugs, whether they have experienced secondary consequences and whether these consequences have been repetitive. While time pressures in the current primary care environment have resulted in attempts to screen for substance abuse using a single screening question (Taj et al., 1998) or using a two-question instrument which screens for alcohol and drug abuse at the same time (Brown et al., 1997), most clinicians still prefer to ask separate questions about alcohol, tobacco and other drugs.

Asking about current or former use of tobacco is a non-threatening way to begin the assessment of substance use. The next step is alcohol screening. The basic alcohol screening approach suggested by the NIAAA includes assessment of quantity and frequency of alcohol consumption and a brief survey of past adverse consequences using the CAGE screening questionnaire (NIAAA, 1995). Quantity and frequency are assessed by asking patients how many days a week they drink alcohol and how many drinks they consume on an average drinking day. One additional question should be used to screen for at-risk binge drinking, either by asking the maximum number of drinks consumed on any given occasion during the past month, or by asking the last time the patient had four or more drinks on one occasion. Since definitions of problem drinking are based on a 'standard drink' of one 12-ounce bottle of beer or wine cooler, one 5-ounce glass of wine or 1.5 ounces of distilled spirits, it is important to ask patients what kind of alcoholic beverages they consume and what a standard drink would be for them. The patient-centered physician may also wish to know the context in which the patient drinks, what beverage the patient prefers, whether he or she drinks alone, when and in what circumstances (parties or at a bar or club).

The CAGE screening exam (Mayfield *et al.*, 1974) consists of four simple questions which evaluate adverse consequences of alcohol consumption and evidence of loss of control. The four items in the screening exam are:

- Cut back: Have you ever felt a need to cut back on your drinking?
- Annoyed: Have people annoyed you by criticizing your drinking?
- Guilty: Have you ever felt bad or guilty about your drinking?
- Eye-opener: Have you ever taken a drink first thing in the morning to steady your nerves or get rid of a hangover?

The CAGE is similar in sensitivity and specificity to the Michigan Alcoholism Screening Test (MAST), a 25-question instrument, and its briefer variations, Brief MAST (BMAST), Short MAST (SMAST) and Veterans' Alcoholism Screening Test (VAST) (Allen *et al.*, 1995), but is much briefer and easier to use. While some studies have shown sensitivity and specificity as high as 94% and 97% respectively (Chan *et al.*, 1994), a review of the literature as a whole shows significant variability in sensitivity and specificity, depending on the population tested (Beresford *et al.*, 1990) (*see* Table 6.1). Other limitations of the CAGE include its focus on the patient's lifetime drinking history rather than current drinking behavior, its relative insensitivity to early problem drinking and some inconsistencies in performance among women and non-Caucasian cultural groups (Volk *et al.*, 1997). Nonetheless, the CAGE has continued to be a practical, useful tool for initial alcoholism screening for more than 20 years. Follow-up questions which clarify any positive responses are extremely useful in aiding in

Table 6.1 Sensitivity and specificity of screening questionnaires

Questionnaire	Sensitivity	Specificity	Reference(s)
CAGE	60–95%	40–95%	Beresford, 1990
CRAFFT	92%	82%	Knight, 1999
TWEAK	79–91%	77–83%	Russell, 1994, 1996
AUDIT	61–96%	62–98%	Allen, 1997; Babor, 1992

test interpretation. At least one study has indicated that the effectiveness of the CAGE with alcoholic patients is much greater if it is preceded by a simple open-ended statement (for example, 'Tell me about your alcohol use'), rather than questions about quantity and frequency of alcohol consumption (Steinweg and Worth, 1993). After asking questions about alcohol use, the clinician may then proceed with questions about recreational drug use, and about any adverse consequences related to such use.

The following interview illustrates how prevention-oriented substance abuse screening can be performed as part of a new patient interview in the primary care setting.

Case study

A 25-year-old schoolteacher presents for a pre-employment physical. He reports no significant past medical or surgical illnesses. He is married with no children, though he and his wife hope to start a family at some point in the next five years. After obtaining a family history, the clinician asks questions related to substance abuse screening.

Clinician: I'd like to ask you a few questions about your use of alcohol and other drugs. Do you smoke, or have you smoked in the past?

Alex: No.

Clinician: Do you drink beer, wine or other alcoholic beverages?

Alex: No, not much.

Clinician: So you do drink a little?

Alex: Well, once a month or so I might go to Happy Hour with some old friends from college, or to a party with my wife and some of our couple friends.

Clinician: When you go out, how much would you drink?

Alex: Oh, two drinks is usually my limit.

Clinician: What about special occasions like New Year's, birthday, anniversary?

Alex: Well, I might drink a little more, but I'm not really much of a drinker.

Clinician: When is the last time that you had four or more drinks on one occasion?

Alex: On New Year's Eve, we went to a party with friends and had champagne. I had four or five glasses, but that's the first time I had done that since college.

Clinician: Have you ever felt the need to cut back on your drinking?

Alex: One time in college I had too much to drink at a party and woke up feeling really sick the next day. That's when I decided two drinks was my limit.

Clinician: Have you ever felt annoyed by others criticizing your drinking?

Alex: Oh no. In fact, when we go out, one of my friends sometimes tries to get me to have another drink with him, but I just say no.

Clinician: Do you ever feel guilty about your drinking?

Alex: No, never had reason to.

Clinician: Ever take a drink in the morning to help get your day started or settle your nerves?

Alex: No. In fact my wife and I make it a policy never to drink before noon.

Clinician: Do you use any recreational drugs like marijuana?
Alex: No. Some of my friends in college tried it, but I wasn't really interested.
Clinician: How about tranquilizers like Valium, Librium or Xanax?
Alex: No, I don't like to take medicine.

The screening interview is now complete. Throughout the interview, the clinician has paid attention to both verbal and non-verbal cues. Alex has answered all of his questions in a very matter-of-fact way, typical of patients who are not experiencing alcohol-related problems. His body language has been relaxed and at ease, and he has not become anxious, fidgety or evasive. The only positive findings in the screening interview were two episodes of binge drinking behavior, one of which occurred during his college days. Although this finding would technically classify him as an at-risk drinker, his risk appears relatively small. The clinician decides to reinforce his healthy patterns of substance use and encourage his observance of the 'safe drinking limits' he himself has set.

Clinician: I want to commend you on using alcohol in a responsible way. Studies indicate that men who drink no more than 14 drinks a week and no more than four drinks per drinking occasion have a very low risk of experiencing alcohol-related problems. It sounds like you have set a very healthy pattern of drinking, no more than two drinks per occasion. I want to encourage you to stick to that limit, since drinking more than that, like you did on New Year's, could significantly increase your risk of having an accident or fall or some other kind of alcohol-related problem.

The clinician has seized the opportunity to utilize Alex's own self-imposed drinking limit as an area of common ground in risk reduction. He uses the information he has given him to identify the kind of situation where he might again be tempted to exceed his limit. Finally, he illustrates possible negative consequences of at-risk drinking by pointing out a typical alcohol-related problem, namely a fall or accident, that might occur in his age group.

Screening of special population groups: adolescence

As in adults, early signs of adolescent substance overuse are subtle and, because experimentation is common, are easily overlooked by parents and physicians. Screening for substance use problems in adolescents is different from screening adults. Not only do fewer physical signs exist, but also the history of use is shorter. Preventive guidelines for adolescent care include screening every adolescent for alcohol or drug use as a part of routine healthcare (Elster and

Kunznets, 1994). Frequently, physicians have not received sufficient education regarding screening techniques and may ask only cursory questions about alcohol or drug use. Starting with more general questions about school, activities or home can help strengthen the patient–doctor relationship which is so central to the patient-centered approach before asking about alcohol or drug use. A promising adolescent screening instrument is the CRAFFT, a brief six-item alcohol- and drug-screening questionnaire that combines items from several other assessment instruments that have proven useful in the past (Knight *et al.*, 1999). These are:

- Car: Have you ever ridden in a car driven by someone (including yourself) who was 'high' or had been using alcohol or drugs?
- Relax: Do you ever use alcohol or drugs to relax, feel better about yourself or to fit in?
- Alone: Do you ever use alcohol or drugs while you are by yourself, alone?
- Forget: Do you ever forget things while using alcohol or drugs?
- Family and Friends: Do your family or friends ever tell you that you should cut down on your drinking or drug use?
- Trouble: Have you ever gotten into trouble while you were using alcohol or drugs?

Each positive answer is scored as one point. A total score of one indicates a need for further assessment and a score of two or more indicates a possible need for a referral to treatment.

Development of trust relationships with adolescents is key to obtaining good historical information, especially regarding sensitive areas such as alcohol or drug use. Sincerity, honesty and questions or statements which demonstrate genuine interest in the individual contribute greatly to the quality of the interview. Confidentiality issues should also be addressed by reassuring patients that information they share in private will not be shared with parents without their permission, unless there is evidence of danger to themselves or others. Parents may be asked to give the care provider a few minutes of privacy to talk with the patient, and be invited to return at the conclusion of the clinical encounter. Health promotion and risk reduction recommendations should be given in a matter-of-fact educational manner that demonstrates respect for the patient's right to make informed choices about the use of psychoactive substances.

Health promotion, risk reduction and screening in women

Because women present to physicians' offices more regularly than male patients, opportunities abound for health promotion, risk reduction, and screening to identify women with substance use problems. Risk reduction regarding alcohol use in pregnancy is a vital responsibility of all primary care providers who treat teens and young adult females. Because of the clear link between alcohol consumption and birth defects, and because there is no clear 'safe limit' for alcohol consumption in pregnancy, clinicians should routinely inform teenage and young adult women of the dangers of alcohol use in pregnancy and encourage abstinence prior to conception and throughout pregnancy.

While all women should be screened for substance abuse problems, certain presenting complaints should alert the clinician to the need for a more careful substance abuse assessment. Well-known alcohol-related physical symptoms include not only problems such as hypertension, epigastric pain and peripheral neuropathy, which are also common in men, but psychiatric complaints such as anxiety and depression. Patient–clinician encounters related to sexually transmitted diseases (STDs) and domestic violence also warrant careful substance abuse screening.

Research evidence that questionnaires such as the CAGE lack sensitivity and specificity in women has led to the development of other screening instruments with greater accuracy (Chan *et al.*, 1993; Russell *et al.*, 1994). Specialized questionnaires such as the TWEAK are facilitating earlier detection of alcohol problems with female patients (Bradley *et al.*, 1998). The TWEAK utilizes the following five questions:

- Tolerance: How many drinks does it take for you to feel high? (≥ 3 indicates tolerance)
- Worried: Have close friends or relatives worried or complained about your drinking in the past year?
- Eye-opener: Do you sometimes take a drink in the morning when you first get up?
- Amnesia (blackouts): Has a friend or family member ever told you things you said or did while you were drinking that you could not remember?
- Kut down: Do you sometimes feel the need to cut down on your drinking?

The TWEAK score is calculated by adding two points for tolerance or worry and one point for each of the other items. Women who exceed established safe drinking limits for women (more than seven drinks per week, or more than three drinks per occasion), who drink in high-risk situations such as pregnancy, or who score two or more points on the TWEAK should undergo a more in-depth substance abuse assessment.

Because of the guilt and shame issues which often accompany substance abuse in women, the clinician must be careful to ask substance abuse-related questions in a non-threatening, empathetic manner. At times, the substance abuse screening interview becomes a dance in which the care provider asks one or two emotionally charged questions (for example, the first two questions of the TWEAK), then withdraws to less threatening questions, only to return later to obtain the necessary historical information. In some cases, numerous office visits may be required before the clinician can draw clear conclusions about the patient's substance use. The continuity experience over time often helps to develop the trust level necessary to explore these painful issues.

Further assessment of patients with positive substance abuse screens

Patients who show evidence of alcohol-related problems or at-risk drinking behaviors on screening require further assessment to determine whether actual alcohol abuse or dependence disorders are present. Again, the presence of denial in many of these patients makes the diagnosis more difficult, and accurate determination of the presence or absence of such disorders requires careful attention. While some authors suggest that primary care providers may simply refer these patients to a chemical-dependency specialist for a more complete evaluation, much as they would refer a patient with a cardiac arrhythmia to a cardiologist for confirmation of the diagnosis and specialized treatment, in many cases this is not necessary. On the contrary, the patient-centered clinician can utilize a variety of additional diagnostic tools while integrating verbal and non-verbal messages and gathering further historical information, following the trail of any subtle clues which emerge in the patient history or interview. Tools which may be useful in creating a more complete picture of the patient's substance use and its possible consequences include the use of written questionnaires, a search for clues using the history and physical examination, laboratory tests or a trial of abstinence or controlled substance use.

Questionnaire screening

One option is to administer a more lengthy substance abuse screening test. Current screening instruments in frequent use in primary care relate almost exclusively to alcohol use, including the MAST (Selzer, 1971a, b), the SMAST (Selzer *et al.*, 1975), the Self Administered Alcohol Screening Test (SAAST) (Swenson and Morse, 1975), and the Alcohol Use Disorders Identification Test (AUDIT) (Saunders *et al.*, 1993b). While the length of these questionnaires (10 to 35 questions) makes them impractical for use in routine screening in most primary care settings, they are quite valuable in helping to provide further information in cases where the extent of alcohol-related problems is unclear. They offer a more extensive survey of potential alcohol-related problems and often provide information which confirms a diagnosis of alcohol abuse or dependency. Many clinicians currently prefer the AUDIT, a 10-question screening tool developed by the World Health Organization (WHO), because its focus is the identification of signs and consequences of problem drinking over the previous 12 months, rather than the entire lifetime (Babor and Grant, 1989). Because it was developed from surveys performed in cultures around the world, the AUDIT is a culturally sensitive instrument with translations which have been validated in several different languages. Two recent reviews of the AUDIT with other screening instruments have shown that the AUDIT had the highest likelihood of both positive and negative prediction of alcohol problems across gender and different ethnic groups (Steinbauer *et al.*, 1998) and shows better correlation with the DSM diagnoses of alcohol abuse and dependence than other instruments (Barry and Fleming, 1993). Paper and pencil formats of the AUDIT, MAST, and SAAST can easily be administered in the clinical setting, even in very busy primary care practices. It should be remembered, however, that these questionnaires do not assess other drug use, and specific questions regarding other potential drugs of abuse must also be asked.

Search for clues from the history and physical exam

Certain presenting complaints may alert the physician to the possibility that the patient has a substance abuse problem. These complaints may relate either to the biomedical (Box 6.1) or psychosocial (Box 6.2) complications of substance abuse. A quick screen of the medical record can be accomplished by reviewing the patient's problem list, presenting complaints on previous visits, hospital discharge summaries or review of systems.

Certain physical findings may also suggest a substance abuse disorder. If the primary drug of abuse is alcohol, the clinician may note mild tremors of the hand or tongue, an odor of alcohol on the breath or use of mouthwash or cologne to disguise its presence, abnormal skin vascularization or conjunctival injection. Simply taking the patient's vital signs may reveal the presence of tachycardia, cardiac arrhythmias such as atrial fibrillation or labile hypertension, while a brief abdominal exam may detect hepatomegaly.

Drugs of abuse other than alcohol may be detected if the patient is presenting signs of withdrawal, such as the yawning, rhinorrhea, diaphoresis, lacrimation and gastrointestinal distress typical of opiate withdrawal or the desperate anxiety, insomnia, sweating and even seizures or delirium associated with

---

Box 6.1   Biomedical problems associated with substance abuse

Emergent or life-threatening

Acute intoxication/overdosage
Withdrawal syndromes
Intracranial bleeding
Seizures
Chest pain in younger patients
Cardiac arrhythmias
Aspiration pneumonitis
Gastrointestinal bleeding
Pancreatitis
Sepsis
Electrolyte/metabolic disorders
Trauma/burns/drowning
Accidents
Pre-term labor
Urgent
Heart failure
Endocarditis
Gastritis
Hepatitis

Peptic ulcer disease
Thrombocytopenia
Fetal toxicity
Non-urgent
Perforated nasal septum
Hypertension
Cardiomyopathy
Cirrhosis/liver failure
Chronic obstructive lung disease
Anemia/marrow suppression
Malnutrition
Neuropathy
Myopathy
Sexual dysfunction
Gynecomastia
Hyperlipidemia
Glucose intolerance
Cancer
HIV

Adapted from Blondell *et al.*, 2000

---

withdrawal from benzodiazepines, especially short-acting medications such as alprazolam. Less obvious clues to the presence of drug abuse disorders may include the odor of marijuana on the patient's clothing, extreme drowsiness or alertness, horizontal or vertical nystagmus, mydriasis, miosis, conjunctival injection or the presence of needle tracks or cutaneous ulcers. Patients seeking to obtain controlled substances from their primary care provider may present with subjective complaints unaccompanied by the usual objective signs of illness, or with dramatic presentations of rather vague symptoms accompanied by demands for a specific narcotic or benzodiazepine medication.

Laboratory tests

Certain laboratory tests may be used to confirm the diagnosis of alcohol or drug problems, or to suggest their presence. The most conclusive of such tests are blood- and breath-alcohol tests and urine drug screens. In certain settings, such as trauma within the emergency department, these tests are routinely obtained.

Box 6.2 Psychosocial problems frequently associated with substance abuse

Psychiatric disorders
Sleep disorders
Depression
Anxiety
Suicide
Memory disorders
Wernicke–Korsakoff syndrome
Dementia
Adjustment disorders
Eating disorders
Family problems
Family dysfunction
Marital problems
Child neglect
Neglect of dependent elders
Domestic violence
Excessive medical care
Social isolation
Social problems
Unemployment
Loss of productivity

Financial problems
Loss of friends
Loss of social support
Economic loss to business
Excessive medical
expenses
Crime
Criminal activity
Robbery/burglary
Embezzlement
Rape
Assault/battery
Homicide
Child abuse/molestation
Spouse abuse
Elder abuse
Driving while intoxicated
Vehicular homicide
Public intoxication

Adapted from Blondell *et al.*, 2000

However, in many primary care settings they are not. The physician should be attentive to issues related to informed consent in obtaining such tests. When informed consent is necessary, the physician may tell patients that he or she wants to be sure they have no serious medical problems associated with drug or alcohol use, and that these tests are routinely done in such cases. Under these circumstances, patients frequently agree to have laboratory tests done. If the patient is resistant, the physician may offer the laboratory tests as a means of the patient convincing the physician that he or she is mistaken about a potential problem.

The most commonly used laboratory tests to substantiate the diagnosis of alcohol problems are the gamma glutamyl transpeptidase (GGT), a liver enzyme which is quite sensitive to alcohol ingestion; the mean corpuscular volume (MCV), a measurement of red blood cell size which increases with chronic alcohol consumption; and the carbohydrate deficient transferrin (CDT), an enzyme related to iron transfer in red blood cells. Elevated GGT levels are 35–54% sensitive and 85% specific for recent heavy alcohol use, and return to normal four to six weeks after cessation of alcohol intake (Rosman and Lieber, 1990). In more severe alcohol problems, other liver tests such as the aspartate amino-transferase (AST) and the alanine aminotransferase (ALT) may also be ele-vated. Increased MCV values occur later in alcohol problems, and they are less sensitive in diagnosing alcohol abuse than serum GGT levels. CDT levels are elevated in patients who drink heavily (over four drinks a day); they are not elevated in other liver diseases. The CDT is more sensitive and specific than the GGT in evaluating problem drinking, especially in male patients under 40 years old (83% sensitive and 89% specific) (Anton and Moak, 1994; Yersin *et al.*, 1995). Using the GGT, MCV and CDT without performing interview screen-ing is discouraged, but these tests can help confirm the diagnosis in suspected problem drinkers.

Trials of abstinence or controlled drinking

Some clinicians utilize a number of self-assessment options for patients to help establish or rule out the presence of a significant alcohol abuse problem. One option is to suggest a trial of abstinence for a period of several weeks. Clinicians who utilize this option should be prepared to manage the emergence of with-drawal symptoms should they occur. Such a trial should be followed by a return visit to the clinician to discuss and interpret the experience. It is important to discuss both whether the patient was able to control his or her drinking behav-ior, and also the emotional consequences of trying to do so. Some patients find that, although they had thought that limiting their consumption would not be difficult, they were mentally preoccupied with the task of remaining abstinent. Others note that their job performance improved or family arguments dimin-ished markedly. While either of these outcomes serves to support the diagnosis of substance dependency, it is important to note that a successful trial of absti-nence does not exclude the diagnosis. On the contrary, the relapse-prevention literature is replete with references to so-called 'white knuckle abstinence', per-iods of abstinence achieved by individuals with substance dependency by means of extreme personal effort, usually accompanied by great personal discomfort.

The authors of *Alcoholics Anonymous*, the guidebook for those involved in AA groups, propose a diagnostic experiment which does not require total absti-nence. It is suggested that patients who are unsure whether they are alcohol-dependent attempt to drink two standard drinks per day for a period of two weeks. Patients with significant problems in controlling alcohol use will find this task virtually impossible to complete, thereby confirming the presence of alcohol dependency.

Finally, some clinicians also encourage patients with unclear diagnoses to attend one or more meetings of AA or NA. In so doing, some patients identify with the experiences of others in the group as they describe the repeated negative consequences of their substance use or their internal struggle to control their use. Again, in such cases, the diagnosis is confirmed and the clinician may proceed with implementation of an appropriate treatment plan.

Conclusion

Major efforts in substance abuse prevention over the past decade have provided us with a much clearer picture of the factors which protect us from substance abuse, as well as those which predispose us towards it. Advances in screening have provided us with instruments tailored to the specific needs of different segments of society. The patient-centered methods provide us with valuable tools which allow us to maximize the application of these developments in the day-to-day practice of health promotion, substance abuse prevention, and early identification of disease.

7

Substance use disorders and the patient–clinician relationship

Michael R Floyd and Ronald S McCord

Editor's introduction

When she was State Treasurer, former Texas Governor Ann Richards made the following remarks to the National Council on Alcoholism:

> 'When I became worried about my drinking and actually got up the courage to talk to my doctor about it, I said, 'You know, I'm really concerned about how much I drink,' and he said, 'How much do you drink?' Gearing up as best I could, I said, 'I drink as much as three really big vodka martinis before dinner.' And the doctor replied, 'Oh well, you don't have to worry about that. I drink that much.' This tells us something about the medical profession and their attitudes' (Richards, 1989).

Implied in this story are the issues of this chapter. Although the apparent dismissal of Governor Richards' concerns may have implications for this physician's knowledge of his own potential problems with alcohol use, the missed communication between two individuals is equally salient. Ann Richards brought with her to the encounter an experience with alcohol and an anxiety about her health and behavior. As she said, it took 'courage' to broach the subject. The clinician, however, failed to appreciate what she was experiencing, missing several significant situational and verbal clues.

This chapter will focus on the patient–clinician relationship, the various ways clinicians and patients communicate throughout the development and maintenance of relationships in the face of substance use disorders. We believe that an awareness of the concepts and skills associated with therapeutic communication and the development and maintenance of relationships are important first steps in assisting healing. Relationships also take into account other factors previously discussed such as culture (Drs Seale and Muramoto, Chapter 1), developmental life stages and gender (Drs Cook and Graham, Chapter 4), as well as family, work and community (Drs Shellenberger and Phelps, Chapter 5).

Overview of the chapter
This chapter is organized into five sections around a clinical story. The first section introduces individuals portrayed in the case: a patient, her husband, family and physician. It provides a framework to illustrate the relational elements described in this chapter.

The second section applies the key concepts of the patient-centered clinical method to specific relationship factors associated with substance use disorders.

The third section describes the personal background of the clinician and patient, examining background elements such as family of origin, work and culture (ethnicity, gender, class, geographical region). It describes important concepts in clinical relationships and demonstrates how these can be applied to substance-abusing individuals.

The fourth section is a dialogue of a clinical encounter between the patient, her husband and doctor. Contained within the dialogue are the thoughts and reflections of the characters, including the clinician's ideas and considerations for advancing a patient-centered approach. Several patient-centered communication methods will be demonstrated, including consideration of the perspectives of gender and ethnicity and skills for reaching common ground.

The fifth section provides a summary and conclusions regarding clinical relationships and patient-centered communications with substance-abusing patients.

Patient–clinician characteristics, context and environment

Case study: the patient
Patty Ellis is a 48-year-old African American wife, mother and nurse who grew up in a predominantly African American town during the early days of desegregation in the South. Patty's memories of growing up are generally positive, amid a tightly knit group of relatives and extended family whose daily activities centered about church fellowship. Her father, Charles, a minister's son, taught at an African American college. Her mother, Isabel, was a nurse, as was her grandmother. Her maternal grandfather Carl, a rail worker, was out of town much of Patty's mother's life and was killed in an alcohol-related automobile crash. Patty's brother, Charles Jr, did well in high school, but despite his ability, quit college. His use of alcohol was a source of dissension and embarrassment within a family of alcohol abstainers. Following military service, Charles Jr lived with his parents, but after

numerous attempts to stop drinking, he moved north and has had very little contact with his family since that time.

Completing a nursing degree in college, Patty married John Ellis, who, following law school, found employment in California, where they have raised three children. Until marriage, Patty adhered to her family's strict prohibition against alcohol consumption. Later, she began drinking a glass or two of wine while accompanying John at work-related entertainment functions. Currently, she is drinking much more and drinking secretly at home after work. She loves John, who, when home, is a caring father to the children, but worries because they seem to be drifting apart from one another.

Patty's older children, Shanika and Richard, secured acceptance into prestigious colleges. Rosalee, her youngest daughter, worries Patty and seems preoccupied with 'friends' whom Patty does not know but whom she suspects use drugs.

Patty is proud to have followed in the footsteps of the accomplished women in her family and maintains a strong identification as a professional nurse. Recent hospital mergers and consolidations have ushered in a time of uncertainty and the threat of transfer from an administrative day position to a rotating night shift. Despite the reassurance of her family, she feels a nagging guilt for not attending her mother's recent illness, being present with the family only at the funeral. She feels blue, overwhelmed at times by what now seems to be a worrisome, hectic pace of life. Lately, her blood pressure has been somewhat elevated, and a trip to her gynecologist resulted in a referral to a family physician for follow-up with this health concern. John has asked to accompany her to this visit. He has told her he is worried about her health and seems to be unusually attentive lately. She thinks it somewhat odd but is grateful for the time he is taking to be with her.

John loves Patty and appreciates her sacrifices: supporting him through law school, moving a great distance from her family of origin, maintaining the household finances and caring for their children. He also has felt guilty for being too engaged in work to help out enough at home.

At first he had been amused, later puzzled and awkward about Patty's alcohol use. Initially, she became more vibrant when she had a glass of wine and he enjoyed her playful wit and social repartee. More recently, these snappy replies have become more cutting, hurtful and loud. He felt increasingly anxious in these settings and either reduced socializing or attended without her. After she protested they were not spending enough time together, and because he felt compelled by his employer to attend, he acquiesced. He suspects her medical problems may be due to alcohol, but when he has brought this topic up, she has become irritated, explaining that she was not at all like her brother, whom she knew was alcoholic. John discussed his concerns with a colleague, who suggested that he attend Al-Anon. He wasn't sure, fearful of the effect of this on Patty's job status. And he feared her anger. He was eager to talk with his wife's doctor and finds himself sitting in the waiting room with her today.

The environment of the patient

The Family in Medical Practice: A Family Systems Primer (Crouch and Roberts, 1987) opens with an illustration by Roy Doty, a cartoon drawing of a woman with a tree sprouting from her head. The branches hold various figures from her family of origin, including a pregnant teenager and a well-dressed, martini-sloshing older male figure. It is no great stretch of the imagination to envision a forest of overarching trees and branches from the heads of both healthcare provider and patient, symbolizing not only family of origin but also environmental and cultural factors that further influence the ways care givers and patients interact. For the patient, these will influence how illness is experienced and perceived. The fact that Patty is a woman, Black, and a nurse all play a role in how she approaches and/or receives help.

Gender

Society has long held ambivalent, negative attitudes about women's use of alcohol (Blume, 1986). Describing gender biases associated with alcoholism, Bissell and Skorina (1987) observed, '. . . it is more acceptable to be a crazy woman or depressed than it is to be a drunk woman', adding, 'alcoholic women are more often prescribed, and become cross-addicted to, prescription drugs than men.' Women often drink in response to a 'one-down' status that is imposed by social roles and then are shamed for being 'unladylike' (Bepko 1991; Gomberg, 1989, 1993). Sensing this discomfort and being influenced by society's mores, clinicians are often reluctant to explore issues that evoke these emotions. Economic limitations, childcare and insurance coverage are also thought to interfere with the provision of appropriate treatment for women (Quinby and Graham, 1993).

Race

Minority women face additional prejudices due to race, culture and language (Quinby and Graham, 1993). Coupled with a history of racism extant in both the North and South is the first-hand memory of a shameful racially motivated incident: the Public Health Service (PHS), under the guise of 'scientific rigor' to determine the long-term effects of antibiotic medication, mistreated some African American patients who languished, untreated, with advanced syphilis. This Tuskegee incident has been seared into the cultural memory of many

Black Americans, but only recently has this influence on African American patients' relationships with the healthcare system been addressed by the dominant society.

Profession

Interpersonal power and role differentiation between professional and economic groups are also factors in forming and maintaining relationships. Historically, nurses have been subordinate to doctors (Fisher, 1995). In the case of Dr Jonas Bucholtz and Patty Ellis, this issue might play out in the roles that doctors and nurses assume with one another. Jonas's attitudes regarding gender, race and professional power differentiation are important, and an openness to the prospect that these factors may be relevant to Patty is even more significant.

Case study: the physician

Jonas Bucholtz is a 55-year-old general internist who grew up in the Midwest on a farm settled by his German immigrant great grandparents during the 1880s. Unlike his brother, who preferred farm life, Jonas preferred academics. He excelled in college and decided to become a doctor. During a medical school rotation one summer, he lived with a community physician, Dr Parrish, and his family in the Deep South. Jonas was used to small, rural towns, but not to poverty and, for the first time, he experienced life as a racial minority.

Jonas's wife's career required employment within a large university. With a significant educational loan debt and limited job prospects for his wife in his hometown, he decided not to return there to practice medicine following residency training.

His experience with alcohol abuse is limited. Although alcohol was a part of his family life, no problems were associated with its use. Focused on his studies, he had little exposure to illegal and 'recreational' drug use. As a medical resident, he felt irritated and disgusted with the relapsing, 'revolving door drunks' who arrived at the emergency room and did his best to avoid these patients. As a practicing physician, he was shocked and bewildered when a colleague became addicted to narcotics. Maintaining personal loyalty with his friend, he also discovered much about addiction that he did not learn through his formal medical training.

The environment of the clinician

The environment of the clinician shapes his or her attitudes and expectations just as it does to patients and clients. These are as varied as the experiences that are unique to each individual. We have chosen to address several of these for illustration purposes.

Gender

Gender plays an important role in patient–clinician interactions. Fisher's (1995) critique of the treatment of women patients by male physicians described medical practices which encouraged women to have unwarranted medical procedures while '... discouraging them to have diagnostic [tests] that were both cost-effective and medically sound'.

Women are seen more frequently in outpatient clinics than men, so it would seem logical that physicians would detect and respond to more problems associated with substance abuse with this group. However, this is not the case. Compared with men, women are less likely to be questioned about alcohol use or to be advised to reduce or stop drinking, and are diagnosed less frequently with an alcohol use disorder (Roman, 1988). On the other hand, they are more likely to be prescribed sedative hypnotic medication, antidepressants and narcotics (Amodei et al., 1996).

Race

Profession and gender have been discussed in the section concerning profession and gender with Patty (being a nurse). Readers are encouraged to consider the issue of race within that discussion.

Profession

Given the importance and time healthcare professionals invest in their careers, it stands to reason that their attitudes would be greatly influenced by these experiences. Clinician attitudes frequently mirror those of society as a whole. These attitudes are reflected by studies finding that alcoholic patients were viewed as management problems rather than individuals needing medical care. Until recently, substance abuse problems were viewed as symptomatic of underlying conflict of developmental delay and not of a chronic primary disease process. A variety of factors are thought to account for ineffective treatment of alcoholic patients: inadequate training, unresolved family of origin addiction issues, personal problems (self-prescribing, negative experiences with addicted patients, rigid clinician personality styles) and fear of loss of collegial support and career advancement (Chappel and Lewis, 1997).

Clinicians have very little formal training in substance abuse. Although the Career Teaching program in ADA (1972–81) was designed for medical faculty development and implementation of substance abuse curricula within medical colleges, the percentage of required coursework and teaching time for substance abuse remains less than 1%. Psychologists, social workers, nurses and other professions were later included in this faculty development through AMERSA, but the Faculty Fellows program, a sequel to the Career Teaching program, was not funded sufficiently to influence the broad-based, interdisciplinary change of 1997. Only Family Practice and Internal Medicine specify training, and the primary care disciplines required supervised management of substance-abusing patients (Chappel and Lewis, 1997).

While training and experience in substance abuse results in optimism among healthcare providers, medical students' experiences with alcohol and other drugs, combined with family members' chemical dependency, may be related to negative attitudes about these patients.

A recent emphasis on impaired physicians has also resulted in some positive changes throughout the profession. Physicians with a previous problem with alcohol and other drugs are more positive about the benefits of an early diagnosis and about accepting and treating these patients. Collegial support is also thought to be a factor associated with more optimistic therapeutic attitudes among clinicians.

Patient-centered communication skills and the patient–clinician relationship

This section will now bring the worlds of Patty and Dr Jonas Bucholtz together. It will begin with an introduction to communication skills designed to demonstrate a patient-centered approach for interacting and for reaching common ground when the worlds of the patient and clinician differ. The section concludes with a review of the factors in the lives of Patty Ellis and Jonas Bucholtz which will influence their relationship.

Essential skills for reaching common ground

Lang *et al.* (1998) describe essential communication skills of a patient-centered clinical interview: rapport building, agenda setting, information management, active listening, addressing feelings and skills in reaching common ground. In the case history of the patient with substance abuse, many of the concepts already noted under the six components of patient-centered medicine will also be paralleled in the six essential skills.

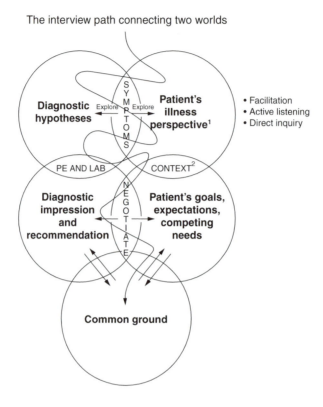

The interview path connecting two worlds

1 Patient illness perspective = explanations, concerns, expectations and impact.
2 Context = patient's personal, family, cultural, work, educational experience and values.

Figure 7.1 A patient-centered model of communication and decision making.

Rapport building

Skills of rapport building are essential when establishing trust and in dealing with perceptions of power. The warm expression of the clinician's interest should include an introduction by name of all the participants in the interaction and statements of personal support where appropriate. This first impression is critical in enhancing the patient–clinician relationship. It is important to actively attend to non-verbal expressions, gestures, facial expressions and contextual clues within the environment, styles of dress and personal possessions that patients may bring into the office.

Agenda setting

Patients are frequently hesitant about discussing their concerns for fear that they will not be considered reasonable or treated seriously (Lang and McCord,

1999). Open-ended questions such as 'What can I do for you today?' followed by non-directed facilitation such as 'Tell me more' and 'What else?' will facilitate the development of a patient agenda. Generally, further exploration should continue until the patient acknowledges that all their issues have been mentioned. Understanding and clarifying Patty's concerns will be important, especially since these concerns are different from those of her husband.

Information management

Clinicians are usually adept in the use of closed-ended questions which objectify symptoms. Other important skills include open-ended approaches, the use of short summaries of the patient's story where appropriate, attentive silence with associated hand or facial gestures, neutral utterances ('uh-huh') and reflecting or echoing the key components of a patient's statement.

Active listening

Introduced by Thomas Gordon (1970), active listening is a means of seeking clarity in understanding those whom clinicians seek to help. Although direct exploration may be utilized to understand their underlying concerns, in our experience patients usually provide clues that, if explored adequately, will more efficiently lead to a full expression of these concerns. A number of common types of clues have been described by Lang *et al.* (2000). The dialogue between Patty, John and Dr Bucholtz will provide examples of some of these clues, such as the expression of feelings, attempts to understand or explain symptoms, speech clues such as repetitive statements, questions or personal stories that link the patient with medical conditions or risk.

Addressing feelings

Strong emotions are often present in clinical situations or are identified during the course of the interview. Dealing with emotions builds rapport, lets patients know of clinician's willingness to help and demonstrates support that can give patients strength to explore difficult issues and consider treatment options associated with substance abuse. Clinicians are encouraged to support emotional expression and to explore thoughts, values and ideas that may contribute to these feelings. Seeing a new doctor and being accompanied by her concerned husband could be an emotionally charged situation for Patty. Uncovering and exploring her husband's concerns, potential grief issues associated with the loss of her mother and a history of alcoholism in the family will also involve strong feelings that may need to be addressed.

Skills in reaching common ground

As Brody (1992) points out in *The Healer's Power*, 'patient-centered primary care extends respect for autonomy into an area seldom, if ever, considered.' Traditionally, autonomy is seen as allowing the patient to choose among therapeutic options offered by physicians. But a patient-centered approach 'forces us to envision a role for autonomy throughout' the patient–clinician interaction. Too often, clinicians rely on a statement of 'the facts', restating their own plan (only louder or more slowly) or use authoritative appeals to convince patients to accept their plan. In a patient-centered approach, the clinician will start with the highest value placed upon the patient's perceptions. Seeking common ground should first come from trying to incorporate suggestions elicited from the patient based upon the patient's perceptions of the problems. Clinician suggestions are necessary. However, these should be tailored to the patient, exploring the feasibility and desirability of the therapeutic options. Sharing power involves the use of creative strategies such as reframing and decision analysis to negotiate differences with the patient's perspective until common ground is reached.

The case we are about to present will involve assessing Patty's readiness to change her behavior in light of the potential effect of alcohol on her health, a concept emphasized in the Transtheoretical Model (Miller and Rollnick, 1991; Prochaska and DiClemente, 1986; Prochaska *et al.*, 1992; Rollnick *et al.*, 1999). Chapter 8 of this book will address this model more fully and demonstrate ways in which communication skills enhance the process of facilitating health behavior change.

Relationship factors with substance-abusing patients

Complex emotional interactions occur in development of the patient–doctor relationship. Stewart *et al.* (1995) have identified six important factors in relationships: power, caring, healing, self-awareness, transference and countertransference, and maintaining realistic expectations. This section will associate these factors with substance use disorders, focusing upon relationship and communication issues that will follow in the clinical dialogue between Patty and Dr Bucholtz.

Power

Clinicians are often frustrated because substance-abusing patients remind them of how little power and control they actually have. Control is also a factor in the lives of patients. In our case example, Patty is ambivalent about becoming aware of the loss of control she has over the effect of alcohol use in her life and feels powerless against the cravings she may experience. She is fearful of discussing the adverse effects that this drug has had on her family relationships and of losing emotional control with Dr Bucholtz, a person she has not yet come to trust. She may have attempted to control her use of alcohol in the past, but failed. Helping her understand that lapses and relapses are a natural part of alcoholism, just as with other chronic diseases such as diabetes, will be an important goal.

As clinicians seek to find common ground with their patients, a fluidity of control is apparent over time. Offering advice prematurely often backfires, especially with an ambivalent patient. Dr Bucholz may believe that an immediate discontinuation of alcohol use is of paramount importance for Patty. However, he may delay pressing for this recommendation until Patty has fully considered the implications of her alcohol use or has attempted a trial of 'cutting back'. He does not ignore or abdicate responsibility for her care; rather, he relinquishes an insistence that she must immediately comply with a particular prescription.

Caring

Francis Peabody's (1984) oft-quoted injunction that 'the secret of the care of the patient is in caring for the patient' is as relevant now as it was when first published in 1927. 'Caring implies the doctor is fully present and engages with the patient. The notion of the detached clinician who keeps a safe emotional distance is replaced by the notion that doctor and patient are interconnected in such a deep way that the doctor can be fully immersed in the concerns of the patient' (Montgomery, 1993). For a busy clinician, it may seem easier to avoid personal involvement than it is to recognize and respond to the substance-abusing patient's unique humanity. Caring clinicians may directly express concern through self-disclosure. This sharing of one's personal experience can be a helpful offering of hope. On the other hand, self disclosures may be harmful in distracting away from the patient's concerns or be interpreted as uncaring and judgmental.

Trust

Trust assumes reliance on the character, ability, strength or truth of someone or something. A trusting relationship with substance-abusing patients is often difficult to achieve, and a clinician's desire for reciprocal trust with a patient may not be realized. This is because recidivism can create a sense of distrust of patients who made previous commitments to treatment. Nevertheless, patients expect clinicians to attend to their welfare, and it is the clinician's responsibility to be constant and focus upon this. Medical realities and consequences compound the difficulty of establishing and maintaining a trusting relationship with substance-abusing patients. It is not easy for a clinician to remain engaged, flexible and open, nor is it for the patient to trust the clinician when things go wrong.

Healing

Curing may involve a permanent change, but healing restores a person's sense of 'coherence, wholeness, and connectedness' (Stephens, 1982). Along with many other professionals, doctors are experienced as 'instruments (agents) of healing.' Balint (2000) asserted that the physician's role in the patient–doctor relationship was like a drug in that it actually has a tangible effect on patient health outcomes.

Self-awareness

Working with substance-abusing patients may create negative feelings and emotions. Trying to keep these out of one's awareness limits personal energy and clinical acumen as clinicians become preoccupied with other things and miss out on important factual and clinical information. 'Mindful' clinicians who tolerate and consider the origins of their emotions may learn to use this awareness on behalf of their substance-abusing patients (Epstein, 1999). Three methods for developing self-awareness include Balint seminars, family of origin groups, and personal self-awareness groups (Epstein, 1993). Personal reflection on literature and the arts is another way for developing self-awareness. Sonya Cashdan and James Turnbull in Chapter 3 of this book offer a variety of media through which clinicians can increase this awareness with substance use disorders, including a movie based on the book *The Doctor* (Rosenbaum, 1988), and the experiences of Dr Martha Morrison in *White Rabbit* (Morrison, 1989).

Transference and countertransference

Transference and countertransference involve projection of feelings, ambivalence or dependency on persons within one's current life and occur within all relationships. In the clinical encounter to follow in the next section of this chapter, Patty transfers the frustration onto her husband, whom she views as being the cause of all of her discontentment. She transfers ambivalent feelings of distrust, shame and guilt on to Dr Bucholtz, whom she expects to judge her harshly in the same way she judged her alcohol-abusing brother. Dr Bucholtz's consideration of transference enhances his capacity to care and provides a therapeutic experience for her.

Countertransference may be displayed through avoiding patients, inattentive listening, misjudging patients' emotions, overidentification with patients, 'enabling' by placing patients in unrealistic, dependent roles or engaging in power struggles. Substance-abusing patients are often aware of clinician ambivalence and perceive this as judgmental or rejecting. Being aware of these incongruities, clinicians reduce conflicting feelings and provide compassionate care.

In the clinical case study to follow, Dr Bucholtz is aware that he has experienced prejudice against substance-abusing patients. However, since his medical colleague was recently treated successfully for a chemical dependency, his attitudes toward substance-abusing patients have changed, leaving him open to addressing these concerns whenever they surface. He has learned to be more patient, attentive and forthright, to develop collaborative, long-term, working relationships with these patients, their families, other care providers and with members of self-help organizations such as AA.

Being realistic

Stewart *et al.* (1995) describe three components of realism in clinical practice: time and timing, accessing resources and team building, and wise stewardship. Effective clinicians need to be able to locate, motivate and promote change while attending to their own personal limitations. Fostering and maintaining clinical resources may involve co-ordinating, co-operating and collaborating as a treatment team member. Changes in the medical system require that clinicians steward the needs of patients while considering healthcare agencies, healthcare system employees and society in general. 'Coping with the growing demands of bureaucracy and its threat to patient-centered care requires constant conscious attention to the realities of the evolving healthcare system. Doctors must ensure that patient-centeredness and the patient–physician relationship do not suffer in the process of making trade-offs' (Stewart *et al.*, 1995).

Many of these relational issues will be illustrated in the clinical case study. Dr Bucholtz will appear to Patty and her husband as non-judgmental, friendly and trustworthy. Power issues could emerge with the professional and gender differences between nurse and physician. Important expectations based on cultural and racial differences could also emerge as an issue of trust, as racism has been and continues to be a concern for patients and providers. Self-awareness, transference and countertransference are also major background issues that could emerge. Will Patty misinterpret her physician's concerns regarding her health and use of alcohol? Can Dr Bucholtz prevent his previous experience with substance-abusing patients from tainting this new patient–doctor relationship? How will Dr Bucholtz realistically manage his time and other resources with Patty and her husband?

The patient–clinician encounter

Applying the patient-centered method to substance use involves consideration of both the disease and the illness experience. From our advance knowledge of the clinical case study, Patty expects her visit to the physician to center on her elevated blood pressure and level of stress. She attributes these conditions to her stress, mood, mother's death, brother's alcohol problem and husband's concerns about her health. John will accompany Patty and be present during at least part of the consultation. He, too, possesses a set of expectations and beliefs along with associated emotions. Initially, the physician will be unaware of these issues and will have the task of addressing both the hypertension and the issues of stress along with the prospect of alcohol abuse or dependency.

As described in the case history and in our anticipation of the patient's expectations, emotions and understanding the whole person is essential to understanding the patient's experience and, as we shall see later, in finding common ground. Patty's gender, cultural and family circumstances influence her experience and beliefs about her illness. Consequently, the clinician will need to pay attention to any information that will illuminate the contextual issues that have influenced Patty and her appreciation of her illness.

Patty and her husband have different perceptions about her alcohol use. If the clinician also becomes concerned that alcohol use is a health issue for Patty, how will he negotiate goals and a treatment plan? In this case, the husband, too, will have expectations about possible treatment options and consequences. Can a plan be skillfully negotiated that will address all concerns?

Patty comes to this physician to address a specific concern, hypertension. Her physician may want to use this and future interactions to address her overall health and consider a broader perspective of illness prevention and health promotion. Patty has emotional reactions which are linked with her family history and does not associate the hypertension with her alcohol use. A non-judgmental, supportive relationship with her physician may provide the opportunity to help her make this connection.

Case study

Dr Jonas Bucholtz, returning from hospital rounds, scans the face sheet of his first case for the afternoon. 'Patricia Ellis, Temp: 98.5, Pulse: 82, BP: 165/114, Smoker: $\frac{1}{2}$ pk q.d., low nicotine brand,' it reads. 'She prefers "Patty",' his office nurse adds, stopping for a moment, raising an eyebrow, a sign Jonas knew might signal the unusual. 'She is an RN at the Medical Center ... her husband asked to stay in with her.'

Dr Bucholtz: [*entering the examination room*] '*Hello, I am Dr Jonas Bucholtz.*'

Patty: '*Hello Dr Bucholtz. Dr Gray set us up with this appointment. I don't know what all the fuss is about. My blood pressure has been up a little bit lately, nothing to get upset about. My husband insisted that I come in today. All this fuss, I just need to relax a bit. My blood pressure has been within the upper limits of normal, generally running about 144/92.*'

Jonas notes that Mrs Ellis's speech is carefully articulated ... the cadence, the vowels, remind him of the time he spent in the rural South before his fourth year of medical school. Yet, her diction is clearly more refined ... The presence of Mr Ellis is interesting, though. While she is knowledgeable, she seems to protest. Perhaps this is a clue to some underlying emotional concern. Jonas sits in anticipative silence, an open gaze toward both Mr and Mrs Ellis, waiting.

John: '*And I am John, Patty's husband.*'

Dr Bucholtz: '*It's a pleasure to meet both of you. How might I be of help to each of you today?*'

John: '*I'm concerned about my wife's blood pressure.*' He has an apprehensive expression on his face.

Dr Bucholtz: [*observing the intonation and facial expression suggestive of underlying emotions, exploring further, looking for clarification*] '*I see ... any particular concern, Mr Ellis?*'

Patty: [*interrupting*] '*I know my pressure was high the other day, but it has only been high for a few weeks, and I am just so wound up with entertaining for John's clients, with our stress.*'

John: '*Do you think that this could be due to stress, Doctor?*'

'Hmm', Jonas thinks, 'a loaded question, I wonder what could be at the bottom of this?' and contemplates the situation. 'The presence of both Mr and Mrs Ellis appears significant – perhaps a clue of an underlying concern. She seems impatient to interrupt and attributes these symptoms to stress, 'our stress,' to be exact. John's affect suggests worry about Patty's blood pressure. He seems to be wondering about stress, but what might lie behind an otherwise innocuous question?' Dr Bucholtz decides to respond to Mr Ellis's clue first.

Dr Bucholtz: '*Mr Ellis, do you think that the increase in blood pressure might be related to stress?*'

John: 'Well yes, Doctor, I am concerned about Patty's reaction to the stress. She lost her mother a few months back. Since then, things have been worse.'
Dr Bucholtz: [following up on the related information suggestive of an emotionally charged situation] 'Things have gotten "worse" . . .'
John: 'Yes, well Dr Bucholtz, I am concerned that Patty is not sleeping well, her blood pressure is up and she . . .' [he pauses].
Patty: 'Now John, you're not going to start up with that now!'
Dr Bucholtz: [recognizes and responds to the emotional clues and addresses both individuals] 'This seems to be an important, but tense topic.'
Patty: 'I'm so mad, I don't know how he could think that! I am not drinking too much. I only have a couple of drinks in the evening when we are not entertaining – just to relax me a bit. There really isn't any harm. Doctor, you know that a little alcohol can actually be beneficial to your health. So, John, you have no basis to think that I have a drinking problem.'

Jonas thinks, 'Is drinking an issue here? I could use the CAGE approach at this point. I already know she is 'annoyed' when someone says something about her drinking. I wonder if she has ever considered 'cutting down'. Suspect she may be in the pre-contemplative stage and not likely to be very motivated at this point to change her drinking behavior. Think I will try to settle things down a bit, first, by addressing her feelings. Perhaps, then, we can establish 'common ground' by agreeing on a health concern.'

Dr Bucholtz: 'This seems upsetting to you, Mrs Ellis. Is this something you would like to talk about right now?'
Patty: 'Yes, I would. I know that John is worried about me, but I just don't believe things are that bad. I think he is worried about nothing.'
Dr Bucholtz: 'It's nice to know he is concerned, but you two disagree on just how serious things are.' [reframing from a position of 'attack' to 'concern']
Patty: 'Exactly.'
John: 'Doctor, I know from the newspaper that alcohol can contribute to high blood pressure. Patty has at least two and sometimes four or more drinks each evening. With her blood pressure, that cannot be good, and her brother has an alcohol problem.'
Patty: 'Well, I don't. I can stop drinking any time; I do not have a problem. I just need to relax. Dr Bucholtz, can you give me something to relax and help me sleep?'

Jonas observes that John is using a problem-solving method for dealing with this issue. He notices that Patty has changed the subject, and he observed the 'repeat' clue ('to relax') along with an intense tone suggesting strong emotions in her question. He considers whether to attend to her request for a sedative or to attempt to segue from John's statement about Patty's alcohol use and blood pressure to an explanation of the effects of alcohol. 'A mini lecture would be much easier right now than having to deal with an angry patient and a husband who thinks I am ignoring his concerns', Jonas thinks. He decides to address the communication issues first and uses reframing to help this couple appreciate his understanding of each other's concerns.

Dr Bucholtz: '*Mr Ellis, you are really worried about Patty* [John nods]. *Mrs Ellis, you accept John's concern and disagree with him about the role that alcohol might play in causing the medical problems you are having. Is that correct?* [Patty and John nod] *I would like to follow up with some questions, Patty. First, though, I want to be clear on the idea that you view your elevated blood pressure as being related to stress and problems sleeping.*'

Patty: '*That is correct. I just know I am not an alcoholic, but I am willing to talk about it.*'

Jonas considers Patty's statement to be a clue as to her thoughts and attitudes about alcohol abuse and makes a mental note to follow up on this at a later time. He decides to assure emotional support before exploring further.

Dr Bucholtz: '*These issues are difficult to discuss, but I am pleased you came in and are willing to consider the kinds of things that can affect your blood pressure. You seem to have some clear ideas about alcohol abuse.*'

John: [having had his primary concerns addressed] '*I think I can go now. I just wanted to make sure that a couple of questions were brought up.*'

Dr Bucholtz proceeds with the interview. Mrs Ellis's past medical history reveals no serious illnesses. Generally, she has enjoyed good health. She had a bilateral tubal ligation following the birth of her third child, a daughter. No other hospitalizations save for normal vaginal childbirth. No allergies. 'Yes,' her appetite had decreased lately, 'No,' she had not lost any weight. He noted that she gave another clue to her ideas of the causality of her symptoms while, during history of GI signs and symptoms, Patty had said, 'It seems like my stomach is always upset. Could it be an ulcer?'. Jonas considers, 'Should I check for more symptoms, or is the time right to ask her directly about her ideas?'. Deciding to explore her clue further, he responds.

Dr Bucholtz: '*You asked whether this could be an ulcer. Tell me your thoughts about that.*'

Patty: '*Yes, well, I am just so wound up with things at home, with entertaining clients of my husband's law firm, with our stress.*'

Dr Bucholtz: '*I see . . . mmm.*' He thinks, 'Another background clue about the family situation and another 'repeat' clue. Patty's ideas about 'stress' really need addressing.'

Patty: [continuing] '*. . . I just can't get John to help out at home. I know that he is busy but I support him with his job. I've exercised in the past, but lately I've been too tied up with work.*'

Dr Bucholtz: '*It must be frustrating . . . Any time you feel calmer?*'

Patty: '*I seem more relaxed when I am entertaining with my husband.*'

Dr Bucholtz: [considering the clue suggested in the comments about her husband and, using non-directed facilitation] '*Tell me more . . .*'

Patty: 'Yes, you know, office parties and the like. And, I like to have a couple of glasses of wine in the evening when we are not entertaining – just to relax me a bit! There really isn't any harm.'

Dr Bucholtz maintains a calm silence, waiting for Patty to continue.

She thinks, 'I hope that he doesn't start on those questions that my gyne-cologist, Dr Gray asked me. The very nerve, asking me how much I drank and if I had ever felt guilty about drinking. He was treating me like I was an alcoholic or something!'

Patty: 'Well, it's mostly at parties with my husband and . . . Doctor, what does this have to do with my blood pressure? And, I know that I cannot be an alcoholic.'

Dr Bucholtz realizes this is another of a series of clues suggestive of denial, and he sees a strong need on the part of the patient to minimize the situation to avoid the strong feelings which she has concerning her use of alcohol. 'She seems to have a very strong need to *not* be alcoholic', he thinks. Jonas seeks to calm Patty using an 'I message', a form of self-disclo-sure, to clarify his inquiry and to help her to understand that he is not blaming her for this situation.

Dr Bucholtz: 'Oh, I see. The reason I seem to be pushing so hard is that I am worried about the potential role that alcohol might play in elevating your blood pressure. You said you know that you cannot be an alcoholic . . .' [He waits.]

Patty knows that alcohol can affect blood pressure. She has worked with what she considers hopeless patients suffering a variety of diseases caused by this drug. Her brother had been in and out of 'rehabilitation' without good results. Yet she never has considered the prospect that her alcohol use could be contributing to her blood pressure problem. She considers drinking an important part of her life and has no desire to discontinue. She feels disconnected from her husband and enjoys the times they spend at his social gatherings.

Patty: 'But it helps me calm down.'

Dr Bucholtz: [hearing this clue about the importance of feeling calm repeated] 'Yes, and that is important for you. I will remember to address this with you as we go on today. What do you think about the possibility that alco-hol may be adversely affecting your blood pressure, perhaps even your stomach problems?'

Patty: 'Maybe so . . . I just need it to help me get to sleep at night.'

Noticing the strong non-verbal clue, Patty's pained, worried face, her eye glistening with a tear, Jonas thinks, 'no reason to ask the CAGE, 'G' for Guilt question . . . she has already answered it.' He responds to what he thinks might be her feelings at this moment while acknowledging her con-cern about not getting restful sleep.

Dr Bucholtz: 'Yes, sleep is important. You also seem worried and a bit dis-couraged.'

Patty tells Jonas about her brother, Charles. Her drinking was nothing like his. Still, she feels ashamed, but relieved when Dr Bucholtz tells her that many people might be embarrassed talking about this and that he can see why this is particularly difficult for her to consider. Jonas attends to Patty's feelings and seeks to offer hope and support.

Dr Bucholtz: 'It must be frightening to imagine that you would end up like your brother. What a hopeless feeling ... [Patty nods]. It takes real courage to talk about these things ... Now that we think about it, you suspect that alcohol might be more harmful to your health than you had realized. But giving up drinking completely is something you really don't want to do at this point.'

As the 30-minute session concludes, Dr Bucholtz and Patty negotiate a plan to explore the role of alcohol in her health and social life. She agrees to monitor her alcohol intake over the next two weeks and to return to the clinic. As they discuss ideas, she suggests that John be included in future planning efforts. She also agrees to speak with a counselor Dr Bucholtz recommends as a means of learning more about the effects of alcohol on her health and life. She is encouraged by Dr Bucholtz's statement of support and commitment to see her regularly. She intends to cut back to no more than two glasses of wine every other day, even if entertaining. Patty expects that she will be successful with this and is hopeful that this is a problem she can overcome. She realizes that she is not to blame for her situation and is relieved that Dr Bucholtz is supportive, and grateful that he is willing to help her.

Substance use disorders and clinician–patient relationships

Summary, conclusions and recommendations

As suggested in Governor Ann Richards' story that opened this chapter, active, sensitive communication is crucial in working with substance-abusing patients. A patient presenting because of questions about her alcohol use is a significant environmental clue. Governor Richards used the affect-laden word 'concerned' when describing the amount she drank. She even emphasized this emotion, saying she was '*really* concerned', and emphasized the amount, 'three *really* big vodka martinis'. Her doctor seemed to realize that 'concerned' may have meant 'worried' but failed to explore her reasons for this concern. He responded from his own experiences with alcohol and attitudes about drinking ('I drink that much') shifting focus away from his patient's experience.

A patient-centered approach offers more subtlety and a deeper relationship with the patient. For example, Patty's attitudes about alcoholism appear to be linked with the frustrating and shame-filled experiences that she had regarding her brother. In addition, the secretiveness associated with her maternal grandfather's probable alcoholism along with the rigid, moralistic, attitudes of her grandmother and parents may have influenced Patty's expectations and emotional state during her introduction to alcohol use. Her family of origin's strong prohibitions against alcohol also limited her exposure to models demonstrating appropriate, responsible moderation in the social use of beverage alcohol. Her experiences, beliefs and attitudes prevented her from being cognizant of the harmful impact of this drug on her psychological, social and physical well-being.

According to the Transtheoretical Model, Patty entered the session in the *pre-contemplative stage*. She was poorly motivated to consider changing her alcohol use. She believed that her difficulty was related to the stresses of coping with work, her daughter's problems and a husband who she feared no longer desired her. With the assistance of her physician, she engaged in a process of gathering information that led her to become more ambivalent about her beliefs (*contemplative stage*). Because her feelings were acknowledged and respected and her concerns were explored, she decided to discuss the benefits and liabilities of drinking alcohol (*decision analysis*) and determined that her use of alcohol was problematic. Among reasons for her ambivalence were a recognition that she was not like her brother and not like the many patients she had seen as a nurse with advanced stages of alcohol problems. Through her involvement with her state professional nursing association, she had some familiarity with a Peer Assistance Program. However, she maintained an uninformed belief that programs of this type were designated exclusively for relapsing, drug-dependent nurses. Her view of success through treatment was diminished further by her brother's difficulties maintaining a successful recovery from alcohol dependency.

This case study describing the dialogue between a patient, her husband and her clinician illustrates many important communication issues involved in working with suspected substance-abusing individuals and their families. First, Dr Bucholtz acknowledged both Patty and her husband. Early in the course of the consultation, he determined their respective concerns, agendas and individual goals for the encounter. He recognized and gave overt statements regarding the existence of strong emotions, then normalized a possible reluctance to discuss difficult issues. Dr Bucholtz used a communication skill called 'reframing' when he directed a statement to John to shift a perception that Patty might have of her husband as being nagging and controlling, to illuminate concern for his wife's health and to let John know that he had appreciated his feelings. Dr Bucholtz repeated this process in the same statement when he advised Mrs Ellis that he heard both sides of her concerns, including a statement that he realized she maintained a specific disagreement regarding her use of alcohol. He verified his impressions through attention to non-verbal feedback from the couple as he was offering his impressions. Dr Bucholtz demonstrated respect for the patient's autonomy and privacy when Mrs Ellis was given the option of exploring these issues at a later time, without her husband being present.

Mrs Ellis's willingness to talk about her problems was enhanced through Dr Bucholtz's non-directive, open-ended approach during the initial phases of the interview. Communication was enhanced as he encouraged Patty to give her history, uninterrupted, through his use of attentive silence and non-directed facilitation statements such as, 'tell me more'. He also made liberal use of important skills such as therapeutic intent, the empathic wording of questions, through educated guesses about how Patty might be feeling and his supportive, respectful manner. As the interview progressed and he gathered more clinical data, Dr Bucholtz continued to use open-ended questions, actively listened to and explored background and emotional clues suggestive of Patty's feelings and ideas about her condition. He communicated compassion and concern by reflecting an empathic appreciation of Patty's non-verbal clues, the glistening, tearful eye and sigh of discouragement.

Before he presented his assessment or a plan of treatment, Dr Bucholtz presented the patient with an understanding of her concerns from her point of view (i.e. the need for improving sleep, stomach problem, reducing stress and lowering blood pressure). Patty acknowledged that these, indeed, were her primary concerns. Jonas then presented his concerns in a non-judgmental manner that was clear and concise. Most importantly, his answer was directly related to the patient's expressed concerns. As a consequence, Patty was more willing to consider alcohol as being one possible contributing factor for her problems. Jonas offered a partnership with her to overcome her problems. Together, they used a decision analysis and 'brainstorming' to arrive at a plan that was acceptable to both parties. This plan included a couple of elements that are especially helpful in working with substance-abusing patients: frequent follow-up and engagement of a social support network. After agreeing to a 'common ground' plan that included a commitment to return to the physician, a recognition that setbacks, while unpleasant, could be dealt with and that Dr Bucholtz would continue to care for her, this initial session was concluded. His stated assurance demonstrates another important aspect of the patient–clinician relationship commitment. Maintaining this attitude and disciplining oneself to constantly focus on the needs of the patient, regardless of vagaries of diagnosis, difficulties of treatment, and uncertainties and unfortunate circumstances of clinical outcomes is critical in all patient care, especially so when chemical abuse and dependency are present (Stewart *et al.*, 1995).

8

Reaching common ground with patients having drug/alcohol problems: defining problems and planning treatment

Jerry Schulz and Michael R Floyd

Editor's introduction

Most clinicians encounter substance-abusing patients. Up to 20% of visits to primary care providers are related to drug and alcohol problems (Bradley, 1994). With these patients being twice as likely to consult them compared to patients without such problems, primary care physicians are in a unique position to identify and help patients with drug and alcohol problems (Rush, 1989). Although clinicians are at times reluctant to directly address this problem, brief interventions are feasible during primary care office visits (Bien et al., 1993). A recent review of brief patient interventions for alcohol and drug problems concluded that primary care physicians can help change the course of harmful drinking, reducing alcohol intake with both alcohol-abusing and alcohol-dependent patients (Fleming et al., 1997). Moreover, many primary care physicians maintain sustained patient relationships and thus have the opportunity over time to address concerns arising out of substance abuse.

The first component of the patient-centered approach emphasizes the importance of understanding the world views of the patient and clinician. The patient's perspective includes explanations, concerns, expectations and awareness of the impact of the illness. The clinician's view emphasizes understanding the patient's problem from a medical-diagnostic perspective. This diagnostic orientation relies on questioning skills to identify the patient's signs and symptoms: observation, history taking, physical examination and the use of various sorts of tests.

The second component, understanding the whole person, was addressed in Chapters 4, 5 and 7 of this book. It involves an exploration of the personal, family and cultural aspects of a patient's life. The third interactive component involves agreeing upon a common understanding of the problem and of a process for change. Reaching 'common ground' often requires the resolution of divergent viewpoints into a plan that incorporates agreement about the nature of the problem as well as the goals, priorities and evaluation of treatment.

This is the second of two chapters addressing patient–clinician interaction. Both chapters emphasize the importance of effective clinical communication skills. Chapter 7 defined elements and challenges involved in developing and maintaining a clinical relationship. Chapter 8 will focus on communication approaches designed to achieve a common understanding and resolution of problems – reaching common ground. Skills involved in agreement on problem definition and negotiating treatment planning are introduced and a clinical case study demonstrates a patient-centered approach for enhancing a patient's motivation to change his or her drinking behavior.

As depicted in Chapter 7, Figure 7.1, the components in the patient-centered method are interactive with the interview following a 'path' connecting the worlds of the clinician and patient. Just as this path 'weaves' back and forth from person to person, it weaves across and between components of the model.

Understanding and linking two world views

The first component of the patient-centered approach involves an interaction between the worlds of the clinician and the patient. The clinician's world focuses on formulating scientific classification and causation of the signs and symptoms observed and reported by the patient. The patient's world is a subjective experience: explanations, concerns, expectations and the impact of the illness on the patient's life.

Throughout this book, we have emphasized the importance of appreciating the patient's perspective. Clinicians also have a medical-diagnostic function that requires an understanding of health problems and physical findings associated with substance use disorders as well as skills necessary to screen for those at risk.

Patients abusing drugs other than alcohol can present with a variety of medical problems. Each drug causes specific signs and symptoms. In Chapter 6, Boxes 6.1 and 6.2 list several physical and psychosocial findings or conditions that should alert the clinician that a patient has an increased risk for a drug or alcohol problem.

Patients who abuse cocaine may develop chest pain caused by vasoconstriction of the coronary arteries. Young patients (<35 years old) with chest pain should be screened for cocaine abuse by doing a urine toxicology screen for benzoylecgonine. Intranasal use of cocaine (snorting) causes rhinorrhea, sinus problems and dental problems. In severe cases, patients may perforate their nasal septum. Cocaine abuse causes seizures and (rarely) intraventricular hemorrhages. A chronic cough (especially if it produces black sputum) may result from crack cocaine abuse. Marijuana abuse should be considered in adolescents experiencing school difficulties, a chronic cough or worsening of asthmatic conditions.

Minor alcohol withdrawal causes tremor, elevated blood pressure and increased heart rate. This might be seen in a patient who is trying to 'look good', by avoiding alcohol before the clinical visit. These individuals frequently try to mask alcohol use with after-shave, perfume, mouthwash or too much makeup.

Diagnostic concerns are emphasized in clinical training and are important, expected requirements for ethical, quality professional care and third-party reimbursement. Overemphasis of these concerns, however, leads to interviews in which the clinician focuses on interpreting the patient's symptoms and statements rather than clarifying the patient's meaning, resulting in conflicts and frustration for both the patient and the clinician. The patient's attempts to express ideas and expectations may be viewed by the clinician as intrusive, leading to avoidance of a problem area, over-reliance on authority-based problem management, or to an adversarial view of the patient.

Case study: the case of Lester

Lester is a 40-year-old White male who comes to a medical clinic to have a prescription refilled for a medication to treat his stomach pain. His previous physician recently retired. Lester is scheduled for a 15-minute appointment, and there are three additional 'work in' patients for the afternoon. According to his chart, Lester had a gastroscopy two years ago that showed acute and chronic gastritis. He continues to have pain that the prescribed medication benefits somewhat. His breath smells of alcohol and he admits that alcohol makes his pain worse. The physical findings and clinical history lead the clinician to suspect that alcohol is contributing to Lester's problems. How shall the clinician proceed on this short visit on a busy afternoon?

An exclusively medical-diagnostic interview might have attended to the diagnosis at the expense of developing a relationship with Lester. Botelho and Novak (1993) describe a six-step model to address a range of behavioral health issues, including alcohol problems. This approach extends from primary prevention with low-risk drinkers to tertiary prevention with alcohol-dependent persons. The first step of this approach uses alcohol risk screening. A positive screen would lead to the second step, assessment to gather further information about a patient's problems. Educating the patient is the third step. Step Four involves assuring that the patient understands the physician's concern and negotiating agreement from the patient's perspective. Steps Five and Six involve negotiated management and follow-up.

Applying the CAGE method for alcohol-risk screening (Ewing, 1984), the clinician would learn that Lester has Cut down on his alcohol use several times throughout the past year and that he gets Annoyed by his wife's constant nagging about his drinking. He would become upset when asked about how much he drinks each day and tell the clinician that he just wants his prescription refilled. The fact that he also has been drinking in the morning of this clinical encounter would also reveal an Eye-opener. These three positive scores on the CAGE suggest a strong likelihood that Lester abuses alcohol and further assessment is appropriate. What is the clinician to do with this information at this point of the interview? There is limited time and the relationship with the patient may have been compromised. Attending to Lester's feelings would take valuable clinician time, yet his frustration and possible anticipation of an adversarial relationship could result in a failure to return to the clinic except in a medical crisis.

Communicating an understanding of the patient's perspective

A patient-centered approach in screening for substance abuse is somewhat different from conventional diagnostic-focused interviews which are more direct and linear. A patient-centered approach is more indirect and subtle, typically occurring throughout the course of the interview, usually with direct reference to the patient's stated or implied concerns. Exploration of the patient's concerns can guide substance abuse screening, reduce resistance, lead to a common understanding of problems and enhance negotiated agreement for behavior change.

Exploring the patient's perspective involves communication skills such as non-directed facilitation, active listening and indirect inquiry. It also requires the ability to 'put first things first'. In the case of Lester, this means investing time and appreciating and addressing his concerns while building rapport and exploring the medical-diagnostic issues. Skills involved in rapport development include the use of positive non-verbal and physical posturing, non-medical social interaction, as well as explicit statements of interest regarding the patient's concerns and life. The clinician needs to communicate a clear understanding of the patient's expectations of the encounter, his agenda, and needs to be sure that this agenda is addressed.

As the clinician develops an understanding of the medical problems using a balance of open-ended and focused closed-ended questions, she will also need to attend to Lester's perspective through direct questioning about his ideas or expectations or through exploration of contextual and personal clues offered throughout the interview. Preoccupation with a diagnostic and clinical decision-making agenda may prevent her from fully appreciating and exploring Lester's perspective. Clinician interruptions that emphasize symptom quantification rather than clarification of the symptoms from the patient's point of view are examples of this ineffectual approach.

Observing, recognizing and exploring verbal and non-verbal expressions of emotions are important, as is attending to other clues about Lester's perspective and health beliefs. Clues (or prompts) are statements, speech patterns or behaviors which carry implied, but not stated, meaning (Lang *et al.*, 2000). There may be a direct statement concerning the illness, or expressions of feelings, or attempts to explain or to understand the illness or symptoms. Other clues include the spontaneous expression of a personal story, repetition of a statement or idea about the illness (Stewart *et al.*, 1995), or evidence of a prolonged internal search such as apparent thought during lengthy silences. Clues might also suggest the patient has an unidentified concern, dissatisfaction or unmet need. Examples of this might include an, 'oh, by the way, doctor' statement, failure to show up for an appointment, a rapid rescheduled appointment or reluctance to accept recommendations (Lang *et al.*, 2000).

Time is a realistic, limiting factor in this initial clinical encounter. The clinician might well choose to focus on Lester's stated concerns (pain relief), seek to develop a personal relationship and secure an agreement to better understand the causes of his problems during a subsequent visit in the near future.

As an introduction to the medical history, the clinician advises Lester of the reasons for asking questions about 'personal habits' such as alcohol or drug use. She emphasizes an interest in the effects of alcohol on his stomach pain or gastritis and begins the discussion by asking what Lester likes about drinking and how it helps him.

A patient-centered approach focuses on Lester's ideas regarding potential causes for his stomach pain. Lester admits that the pain is made worse by alcohol ingestion. This fact provides a path that begins with his experience and explores his beliefs about his stomach pain and his use of alcohol. Exploring these ideas, the clinician discovers that Lester believes that alcohol helps him to relax and socialize. The clinician gathers important diagnostic information using Lester's own words in follow-up questions such as, 'About how many drinks do you have when you want to relax?' or, 'When you socialize, on an average, how many drinks do you have?'. Other patient clues might afford the clinician the opportunity to follow up with questions related to loss of control, tolerance or binge drinking. When Lester begins talking about his wife's concerns, the clinician might inquire about possible blackouts by asking, 'Has there been a time when your wife nagged you about things she said you did but you can't remember?'.

Lester reports that he drinks three to four alcoholic beverages almost every day. Over the past month, he 'celebrated' several times, consuming about 12 bottles of beer on these occasions. This occurs one to two times a month. He reports that at times he cannot remember what he did after these drinking sessions. After an arrest for driving under the influence of alcohol (DWI/DUI) a year ago, he cut down on his drinking. Once the legal problems settled, he resumed his previous drinking pattern. His wife nags about his drinking and he feels guilty about missing several of his son's baseball games. Occasionally, when he has had a 'bad night', he has a beer or two the next morning to help him feel better. Lester's father died of cirrhosis of the liver. Lester denies any other drug use.

The physical examination reveals that Lester's liver is slightly enlarged and tender, his blood pressure is 145/98, and his resting heart rate is 88. He seems to have a slight tremor and he smells of alcohol. When asked about this, he responds that he had a 'business lunch' before the clinic visit.

Agreeing that it is important to find out causes of his discomfort enhances Lester's willingness to allow for the initiation of diagnostic tests that also might make it easier for him to appreciate the causal relationship between alcohol and physical dysfunction. Laboratory tests could be initiated before Lester leaves the office, provided there is time, but it is important that he recognizes the potential benefits and agrees to this. Lab work would include a set of liver function tests, GGT and a complete blood count (CBC) to look for any elevation in the MCV. This approach has brought together a medical-diagnostic perspective that takes into account the essential physical findings, associated symptoms, screening and laboratory tests with the patient's perspective. Since he smells of alcohol, determining his blood alcohol level (BAL) can be useful. Negotiating this action is ethically sensitive and important in establishing and maintaining a trusting relationship with Lester. A BAL that is significantly out of proportion to his level of intoxication would provide evidence of tolerance. He could be advised that you plan to check the BAL to determine 'how his body responds to his drinking during the business lunch'.

We have seen the clinician use many of the basic skills necessary for negotiating a common understanding of Lester's problems. Using effective communication skills, she has elicited an understanding of his illness perspective and health beliefs. She also has formulated a basic understanding of his medical problems and initiated steps toward further evaluation. The clinician refills Lester's prescription with enough medicine to last until next week when he has been scheduled for a comprehensive visit. In the interim the blood tests arrive, showing Lester has an MCV of 102 (normal up to 99) and a GGT three times normal. His AST and ALT are at the upper limits of normal.

Agreeing upon a common understanding: reconciling clinical impressions with patient goals, expectations and competing needs

As a diagnostic hypothesis is formulated and the patient's illness perspective is explored, the second phase of the patient–clinician interaction continues. This phase involves the presentation of a clinical diagnostic impression and associated recommendations with a patient. The experience of substance abuse and addiction involves a complex set of competing needs within the patient which are expressed directly or indirectly in the clinical encounter. Consequently, this phase often involves an extended process of negotiation and inquiry into the goals and expectations of substance-abusing patients. This process is facilitated when the clinician has fully explored the patient's illness perspective, particularly feelings and beliefs associated with the effects of alcohol/other drugs, causation and expectations about change.

The first step in reaching common ground is defining the problem, clarifying and resolving differences between the clinician's and the patient's points of view. The clinician is responsible for clearly and directly offering an accurate diagnostic impression that is understandable to the patient while remaining alert for and addressing the patient's goals, expectations and competing needs as these arise. This process involves delineating points of agreement and disagreement between the clinician and the patient, identifying priorities and areas where change is needed and assessing the patient's readiness to change. Sometimes clinicians and patients 'agree to disagree' about the presence of a drinking or drug problem, but decide to follow-up on this concern at a particular time in the future. The clinician needs a realistic appraisal of the clinical situation and knowledge of the options for treatment. Clinical communication skills needed in this negotiation include the ability to provide information about the problem and suggestions for change, to use collaborative speech, to check for agreement and feasibility and to establish specific roles and responsibilities for both the clinician and the patient.

Assessing readiness to change

The Transtheoretical Model incorporates many therapeutic methods for understanding intentional behavioral change. It addresses motivation and focuses on specific interventions or skills to be offered at appropriate moments (stages) in which change is most likely to occur (Miller and Rollnick, 1991; Prochaska and DiClemente, 1986; Prochaska *et al.*, 1992; Rollnick *et al.*, 1999). This approach, the basis of Motivational Enhancement Therapy, emphasizes the application of clinical responses that are appropriate for the patient's willingness to initiate a life change rather than the clinician's ability to diagnose and prescribe a treatment plan (Rollnick *et al.*, 1992). This is considered a client-centered method because the client is addressed at his or her particular level of motivation or readiness to change. The therapeutic skills used in each stage are specific for helping to motivate clients to change from one stage to another. Facilitating change requires clinician competence with communication, negotiation, and psychotherapeutic skills. Rather than characterize a substance-abusing patient as resistant or in denial, the therapeutic goal is to facilitate stage-specific change, leading toward action in achieving and maintaining health-related behavior.

A patient in the *precontemplative stage* would not perceive a relationship between alcohol consumption and gastritis and would not be internally motivated to consider changing alcohol use. A *contemplative stage* patient, on the other hand, considering yet ambivalent about behavior change, might be helped from discussions about the potential benefits and risks of continuing alcohol abuse. This discussion might lead to a decision to move toward the *preparation* stage. Progressing from preparation for behavior change, someone in the *action stage* would benefit from clinician encouragement for initiating change and someone in the *maintenance stage* would benefit from continued reinforcement for these changes.

A spiral or a 'wheeled' model, this approach accommodates an understanding of patients who move in and out of various stages of change (DiClemente and Prochaska, 1998; Prochaska and DiClemente, 1983). For example, an individual may move from an action stage into relapse and become pre-contemplative about change. Or, he or she might move from relapse into a preparation stage in which he or she would be seeking to remove obstacles that may have prevented successful maintenance of a desired health behavior. Clinical approaches employed are based on the patient's specific stage of change, including, in the case of substance-abusing patients, relapse recovery. Basing interventions on a particular stage of change, the clinician can employ a strategy that will avoid antagonizing and may eventually help the patient move to the next stage, markedly improving the likelihood of eventually correcting the problem.

Box 8.1   Stages of change

1   **Pre-contemplation**: relationship between problem and alcohol use not appreciated. Patient has not considered change within six months
2   **Contemplation**: considering change, patient remains ambivalent about a time of initiation and method

3 **Preparation** (determination): patient acquiring ideas about change and has determined a date to initiate this
4 **Action**: patient actively initiating actions leading toward long-term behavior and lifestyle change
5 **Maintenance/Relapse**: patient needs encouragement to maintain lifestyle change or needs to be encouraged to return to a contemplative or preparation stage.

During the initial visit, the clinician determined that Lester was in the *precontemplative stage*. He cut back on his drinking about a year or so prior to the initial visit, but has not considered cutting back or quitting alcohol for the past six months. The clinician also initiated an assessment of the severity of Lester's alcohol problem through a detailed history, physical examination and laboratory tests. Important historical clues to the diagnosis included a history of blackouts, tolerance changes, withdrawal symptoms, a positive family history of alcoholism and marital conflict. Other important diagnostic features might have included preoccupation with drug/alcohol use as well as secondary problems such as legal, health, work, financial or other family consequences.

Pre-contemplative patients do not realize a problem exists, are frequently unwilling to discuss the problem and not receptive to recommendations or suggestions concerning their drug/alcohol use. Trying to refer such a patient for substance abuse treatment will often antagonize, increase resistance to change and disrupt a positive patient–clinician relationship. The primary therapeutic role of the clinician of a pre-contemplative patient is to maintain a positive relationship while encouraging the patient to risk becoming unsure or ambivalent with regard to their drinking beliefs, i.e. to become contemplative.

Patients who are in a contemplation stage are generally aware that their problems may be caused by drugs/alcohol, but are ambivalent about deciding to change. If questioned empathically, they are often willing to discuss the dysfunction caused by their substance use. The role of the clinician with contemplative patients is to explore reasons for quitting and for continuing drinking or drugging. One technique that has proven useful in resolving this ambivalence is the 'decision analysis' which involves systematic exploration of ideas and issues that might maintain problem health behavior. Clinicians lead patients in discussing the things they gain and/or lose from continuing their current drinking pattern. This discussion is then expanded to list things they would lose or gain from discontinuing these patterns (Botelho, 1992).

Patients in the preparation stage realize they have a problem with drugs and/or alcohol and are just beginning to think about ways to remedy the problem. They are likely to be receptive to options that will help them deal with the problem. Patients who are in the action phase are very open to clinicians' suggestions and more commonly follow through with treatment recommendations, especially if those recommendations are the result of negotiated planning between the clinician and the patient.

Finding common ground with substance-abusing patients

Most clinicians are familiar with situations in which there is disagreement, where the worlds of the alcohol-abusing patient and the clinician diverge. Reaching common ground with these patients, finding ways of agreeing upon the nature and treatment of the problem, is a clinical challenge. This process is one of the features that distinguishes the patient-centered clinical approach from a 'diagnose and treat' approach or from passive ineptitude.

The initial clinical task is to assure an understanding of areas of agreement and disagreement. Clinicians need to link their concerns about health outcomes with issues and problems that substance-abusing patients find relevant and important. This requires that clinicians effectively communicate an understanding of the patient's perspective and health beliefs while insuring that patients understand and appreciate how complex biopsychosocial problems and medical sequelae directly affect them.

Many substance-abusing patients have a variety of health problems that complicate communication efforts to reach common ground. Years of substance abuse may have led to impaired cognitive capacity. Persons currently under the influence of mood-altering drugs may be unable to attend to the clinician's concerns or fully appreciate the severity of their condition. Psychological resistance or fears of failure may also play a role in diminishing effective communication necessary for reaching common ground.

It is important for the clinician to point out areas of mutual agreement and disagreement regarding substance abuse issues in an explicit, yet non-judgmental collaborative manner. As a general rule when areas of disagreement exist, clinicians are encouraged, at least initially, to avoid behaving in ways that might impede future negotiation. Obstacles to negotiation include the use of scare tactics or overemphasis of morbidity and mortality, the risks and dangers of substance abuse. Other 'road blocks' include moralizing, argument, clinician defensiveness and disregard of the patient's ideas.

Suspecting or anticipating disagreement, some clinicians act as though their patients cannot hear or do not understand them. Examples of ineffectual methods to convince the patient include restating the clinician's original position (perhaps more loudly or slowly), using personal or 'expert authority-based' appeals that disregard the patient's perspective, or becoming allied against the patient when family members or other concerned persons are involved.

Agreeing upon a common plan: development, implementation, 'trouble shooting' and agreement

Effective negotiation strategies

The negotiation process involves an exploration of differing points of view when considering treatment alternatives. This would include a discussion about expectations concerning roles and responsibilities of both the patient and the clinician. The clinician might play several different roles such as one who possesses expert knowledge and skill, offers responsible care, facilitates optimal health outcomes and focuses on the welfare of the patient. By being an active participant in this process, the patient is empowered to assume more responsibility in implementing a treatment plan. While this process may feel cumbersome, perhaps even frustrating to the clinician, common ground, once successfully established, increases the likelihood for successful implementation of a therapeutic plan.

The most important, yet fundamental, negotiation skill is that which seeks a better understanding of the patient's point of view. This can be achieved by revisiting an earlier portion of the encounter, perhaps following up on clues suggestive of resistance, or 're-checking' the clinician's understanding of the patient's ideas, concerns, and/or expectations. Fisher and Ury (1983) offer a number of strategies that are helpful in effective negotiation. A primary strategy is an admonition to remain focused on the patient's and clinician's interests and concerns, not positions to be defended. Basic tactics suggested by these authors include focusing on the problem rather than the patient, generating a variety of possible solutions before assessing and deciding upon a plan, and agreeing upon verifiable, objective criteria to assess a plan.

Other important concepts for developing treatment plans include: tailoring the plan to the patient (identification of intrinsic and extrinsic motivators), addressing potential adherence obstacles, identifying short-, intermediate-, and long-term goals; making sure the patient has a sense of control; being realistic about abilities and outcomes; keeping it simple by being explicit about 'who does what, when, where, and how'; implementing complex plans incrementally; assuring the patient's explicit commitment; engaging significant others in the life of the patient; evaluating effectiveness of the plan at follow-up visits and offering clinician support/encouragement.

A variety of methods for negotiation such as brainstorming, therapeutic compromise, criteria setting, decision analysis and reframing can be employed in developing a treatment plan.

Brainstorming

Brainstorming is a method in which participants generate ideas to solve a problem. Patients and clinicians list as many ideas as possible without evaluating any of them. Evaluation or determining feasibility is the second part of a decision-making process.

Compromise

Clinicians and patients occasionally agree on a plan that takes some ideas from each point of view and may be willing to 'settle' for part of a devised plan or outcome. An example of this 'meeting in the middle,' might be an agreement that a patient may take a medicine at a less than optimal time to accommodate a patient concern. *Quid pro quo* is a variation of compromise in which both the patient and clinician agree to do something in return for another's actions ('You do this and I will do that').

Criteria setting

Criteria setting involves decision-making based on the use of some objective standard or condition determined by clinicians and patients. For example, patients may agree to enter an inpatient treatment center if their attempts to control their drinking on their own fail over the next three months.

Decision analysis

It is often helpful to engage patients in a dialogue by first encouraging them to consider the things they enjoy about alcohol. This negotiation technique is called *decision analysis* or using a 'decision balance' (Botelho, 1992). By encouraging patients to list the positive reasons for using alcohol or drugs, clinicians demonstrate interest in understanding the reasons patients are reluctant to alter or to give up the use of alcohol and/or drugs.

Reframing

Reframing is a clinical skill that seeks to shift the focus of a position or statement in a direction that works toward greater understanding and the achievement of a common goal. There are many different methods for reframing a patient's statement, the clinical situation or a conflict.

> Pre-contemplative patients frequently move into the contemplation stage when they learn about the particular problems that alcohol or drugs cause

in their lives. If present, abnormal laboratory tests can be used as objective criteria of alcohol damage to help patients appreciate the physical consequences of drug/alcohol abuse. Lester and his clinician discuss the relationship between his alcohol use and gastritis. Specifying social events such as failing to attend his son's ball games, the clinician helps him appreciate adverse social and family consequences of his drinking. The clinician is careful in attending to Lester's emotions, exploring and addressing expressions of excessive shame and guilt. This is particularly relevant since he feels quite guilty for disrupting family activities. The clinician uses **emotional reframing** to help Lester realize that his feelings of guilt may be the result of his level of care and commitment for his son and of the high standards he expects of himself as a father.

During their discussion, Lester agrees that alcohol is contributing to his physical and family problems. Should he have refused to consider these problems, his clinician was prepared to 'keep the door open', schedule a return visit to reassess his gastritis or other medical problems, and to look for opportunities to explore his reluctance at a later time.

At the point of the second office visit, the clinician believes that Lester has significant problems associated with his alcohol use and that he is likely to be alcohol-dependent. She thinks he is in the contemplation stage of change, but realizes that pressing him toward an action stage or toward her treatment preference, abstinence, would likely be counterproductive, perhaps harmful to the patient–clinician relationship.

Together, Lester and his clinician 'brainstorm' a list of possible solutions for each of the problems they identified: physical (stomach and liver function), social (arrest for driving while intoxicated) and family (nagging wife and guilt about relationship with son). In addition to helping with social and psychological adjustment, the clinician wants to reduce the harmful physical effects of chronic alcohol use, including withdrawal syndrome that might accompany changes in his drinking pattern. Lester's position is that he enjoys using alcohol with work colleagues. His interest is to be able to relax and socialize after work.

His clinician prefers that Lester become abstinent. One of her 'brainstorming' ideas was that Lester could attend AA meetings (helpful tips in referring patients to a 12-step program are discussed later in this chapter) or a formal drug/alcohol treatment program. She also suggests that referral to a mental health professional might be beneficial. However, she is willing to **compromise** for two months and together they will carefully observe Lester's stomach symptoms and laboratory findings (**criteria setting**).

Lester thinks that he can cut back if he 'tries harder'. His clinician reviews his history, determines that he has not experienced seizures or other severe withdrawal symptoms in the past, provides him a list of the signs and symptoms of withdrawal, and advises that he call or seek immediate medical care if he experiences these. He is willing to monitor his alcohol use to see if his medical problems improve, to make a list of the positives and negatives for using alcohol, to enlist the help of his family, to not drink and drive, and to follow up in two weeks.

While he is unwilling to seek counseling with his spouse, he is willing to involve her in the next visit with this clinician. Depending on the concerns his spouse and son have at the next visit, the clinician might recommend that they consider attending a 12-step program such as Al-anon or Al-ateen. In cases in which the family member presents to the clinician, but the substance-abusing person is unwilling to seek help, the family might consider receiving counseling and/or participating in a formal intervention. Carefully planned, formal interventions are typically conducted with the assistance of professionals who aid the addicted person to become aware of the consequences of their behavior and encourage them to seek help (**decision analysis**).

On his third visit to the clinic, Lester brings the following list of the positives and negatives for his drinking (Box 8.2).

Box 8.2 Positive and negative aspects of drinking

Positive reasons
I like the taste of beer and wine
It helps me relax
I can socialize better
I work hard and deserve to have some fun with the fellows at the bar

Negative reasons
It is damaging my liver
I miss a lot of the family activities
The DWI cost a lot of money

While he is ambivalent about abstinence as a treatment goal, Lester is beginning to consider more of the consequences of his alcohol use. The clinician supports him by acknowledging what a positive step it is for him to come in for the follow-up visit and to complete his list.

His wife does not attend this session and the clinician seeks to understand Lester's ideas about this. He reports that he is not successful in cutting back on his drinking. The clinician suggests that Lester considers referral to a treatment program, but he becomes upset and states the clinician 'just doesn't understand'. She follows up on this clue, and he insists that his drinking is not that serious a problem for him. She reaffirms her desire to help. After they review the reasons he wants to drink, she asks him to recall the health concerns expressed at an earlier session. Lester adamantly maintains a goal of cutting down on his drinking, but agrees to set criteria for 'safer' alcohol use and contracts to average no more than two drinks each day and no more than four drinks on any given occasion. He agrees to accept more intensive help if this plan fails. She writes this plan on to his medical record. Lester agrees to come back in a month. The clinician tells Lester that she hopes he will be successful and that she is there to help over the long haul.

On the return visit, Lester continues to report stomach distress, and his lab work has not changed appreciably. He says that he cut down 'most of the time,' but admits that on one weekend he drank several six-packs of beer and had a blackout. During a discussion regarding the guidelines, Lester spontaneously states, 'But, I am not a drunk!'

Labels can have a negative effect on patients' willingness to accept help and to acknowledge the problems caused by drugs/alcohol. Clinicians are encouraged to take particular care to understand the meaning of affect-laden terms such as 'drunk' or 'alcoholic'. This might provide an opportunity to educate about the fallacy of stereotyping patients with drug/alcohol problems, that alcoholism is a disease that can be treated just like any other disease such as diabetes or high blood pressure. Reframing drug/alcohol addiction as a disease can help patients have less guilt and shame about their addiction. Too much guilt or shame can lead the patient to feel hopeless.

Hearing this clue ('I am not a drunk!') Lester's clinician asks him to tell her more about this idea. He tells of his despair and disgust, remembering his now-deceased alcoholic father, who left the home when Lester was young. Following up on Lester's clue underscores the importance of continuing to listen and responding to patient ideas throughout all phases of treatment. Lester confides that he does not know what to do. The clinician seeks clarification and learns that Lester believes that he may fare better trying to quit drinking completely, but that he fears that he just cannot do it. He is now in a preparation stage for a goal of abstinence and wants help understanding his options. Continuing a dialogue initiated in the second visit, the clinician asks Lester what he thinks the best plan would be for him. He thinks he needs some type of formal help but does not know what is available. Being aware of local treatment options, she suggests that Lester enter an inpatient treatment program. Lester states that he does not have any coverage on his insurance for inpatient alcohol treatment and cannot afford to be away from work.

Compromising, and using *quid pro quo*, the clinician agrees to provide medication for outpatient alcohol detoxification if he will agree to go to an outpatient treatment program. Outpatient drug/alcohol detoxification is both cost-effective and safe if certain guidelines are followed (Fleming, 1991).

Box 8.3   Outpatient detoxification criteria

Medical criteria
Absence of serious medical problems
No history of recent trauma
No history of drug withdrawal-induced delirium or psychosis
No history of withdrawal seizures
Patient can be detoxified with 300 mg of chlordiazepoxide or less

Abstinence criteria
Patient agrees to abstinence
Patient agrees to random testing
Patient agrees to take part in a treatment program

Psychosocial criteria
Patient has social support of sober family or friends
Pre-existing relationship with the physician

Physician criteria
Patient able to see physician daily until the withdrawal symptoms subside
Physician has expertise in recognizing and treating withdrawal symptoms

---

Some younger, healthier patients with no previous history of severe withdrawal problems or any complicating medical problem are able to detoxify themselves from alcohol with no medication. The ASAM (ASAM, PPC–2R, 2001) has developed criteria to help decide the appropriate level of care for drug/alcohol treatment. A recent meta-analysis reported that benzodiazepines are the most effective detoxification medications (Mayo-Smith, 1998). To avoid oversedation, detoxification treatment should be individualized and symptom triggered (Saitz *et al.*, 1994).

Lester plans to take the weekend off to detoxify using the chlordiazepoxide prescribed by his physician, to initiate the comprehensive outpatient treatment program at the beginning of the week, and to be seen again in the clinic before the end of the following week. He balks at the clinician's suggestion that he attend an AA meeting, saying that he hates groups and doesn't think he would do very well in AA. He is also concerned that someone might see him at the meeting. She uses active listening to explore his ideas and fears before proceeding.

It is important for clinicians to understand the basic principles of 12-step pro-grams so they can make successful referrals. One of the best ways to become familiar with AA is to attend a meeting. Some 'closed' meetings (for alcoholics only) allow clinicians to attend with a member of the group or contact the group beforehand. Anyone can go to an 'open' AA meeting. Literature is available for interested clinicians through AA World Services in New York. It is also helpful for clinicians to maintain a current listing of local 12-step meetings to give to interested patients. Most cities list AA, Al-anon, and other self-help groups in phone directories, and newspaper announcements often list meeting loca-tions, dates and times. One effective way to help patients to attend 12-step meetings is to make a direct referral to someone in the program and help the patient have personal contact with someone in recovery. Sisson and Mallams (1981) found that attendance in AA by newly-diagnosed alcoholics was signif-icantly greater when these persons were put into direct contact with an AA member rather than being encouraged to attend a specific meeting. Most medi-cal practices will have some patients who are in a 12-step recovery program, and frequently these patients will be very willing to help a newcomer to get to a meeting.

> The clinician addresses Lester's concerns and learns of his fears about talking in the group. He is advised about the format of the AA meeting and informed he can attend without participating in the discussion (just say you 'pass'). Some patients are reluctant to attend 12-step programs because they believe that the meetings are religious and God-oriented. Twelve-step programs are spiritually-based, but do not require a mem-ber to believe in God. *Alcoholics Anonymous*, the AA 'Big Book', contains a chapter for agnostics (Chapter 4, 'We Agnostics'), and clinicians are en-couraged to familiarize themselves with this. Another misconception that many patients have is that they need to be sober to attend AA. They can be informed that one of the 12 traditions of AA is that 'The only requirement for membership is a *desire* to stop drinking'. Once his concerns have been addressed, Lester agrees for the clinician to contact one of her recovering patients, and to go with this patient to an AA meeting.
>
> As agreed, Lester attends the comprehensive outpatient program. The program also offers special help for his wife and son through separate and joint family sessions. Several weeks after completing treatment he returns to see his clinician for a follow-up visit. He thanks her profusely for helping to turn his life around. He says that he has never felt so good, has quit smoking, gone on a diet, started an exercise program, planned a second honeymoon and has volunteered to be on several committees in his church. He tells the clinician his stomach is fine now and he does not need any medication. Experienced clinicians are alert for what occasionally

occurs at this stage: Lester is on a 'pink cloud' after completing a drug/alcohol rehabilitation program. Trying to make too many changes early in recovery can lead to frustration and relapse. One of the AA aphorisms is 'Easy does it'. Lester's clinician should explore his exuberance, perhaps encouraging him to focus on one or two changes at a time, especially in early sobriety. He needs to be encouraged to remember that his number one priority is staying sober and that by trying to do too many things, he is jeopardizing his sobriety.

Unfortunately, Lester ignores her advice and continues with his frantic pace. Two months later, the pharmacy calls and asks about a refill on his stomach medicine prescription. The clinician then realizes that he did not show up for his last appointment. The prescription is refilled and Lester is called to arrange a follow-up visit. The call is met with anger and resistance to coming in because he is 'too busy'. Reluctantly Lester agrees to come in.

During the clinic visit, when he is asked about his meetings, Lester looks down and says he really 'didn't get into them'. He attended a few meetings after treatment but then got too busy and stopped. The clinician asks how his sobriety is going, and he says 'Fine!' When she explores this further, he reports that he has started drinking again, even more heavily than when he originally quit.

It is important for clinicians to remember that drug and alcohol addiction is a chronic, often relapsing condition. For most patients, relapses '. . . are almost inevitable and become part of the process of working toward life-long change'. Ideally, patients are educated about relapse early in treatment and develop a relapse prevention plan. Rapid, significant, negative medical and social consequences often follow relapse. Empathic inquiry is necessary when addressing this situation. Feeling considerable guilt and shame, relapsing patients are very reluctant to return to see their clinician.

This is an example of how understanding the 'Stages of change' *relapse stage* can facilitate therapeutic interaction. As they explore and understand a patient's health beliefs and ideas concerning causation and locus of control, clinicians can offer specific cognitive-behavioral suggestions for skill development or other changes. It is important that patients be helped to determine what led up to the relapse and how it might be prevented in the future. Relapses are unfortunate, but are best viewed as an opportunity to learn, not as examples of failure.

Using active listening, the clinician attends to Lester's discordant tone, exploring the possible meaning of underlying feelings associated with the statement that he was doing 'Fine!' She reframes the relapse to motivate and re-engage Lester in the change process and discusses ideas to prevent a recurrence through using another **brainstorming** activity. She suggests that he re-establish contact with friends who are 'in recovery' and that he attend an abbreviated treatment program. Lester has heard of a new medicine, naltrexone, and thinks he would like to try it.

Medications

The use of naltrexone to treat alcohol dependence was first reported by Volpicelli *et al.* (1992). The endogenous opioid neurotransmitter system appears to be part of the craving experienced by alcohol-dependent patients. This system also appears to be part of the positive reinforcing effect of alcohol. When an alcohol-dependent patient drinks, naltrexone blocks the reinforcing effect of alcohol, and the patient does not experience the usual pleasure and euphoria. Naltrexone should not be used with opioid-dependent patients, or those with acute hepatitis or liver failure. It is most efficacious when used in conjunction with other treatment modalities, such as supportive therapy and coping skills training. The most common side effects of naltrexone are nausea (10%), headache (7%), dizziness (4%), nervousness (4%), fatigue (4%) and insomnia (3%).

Acamprosate has been used in Europe to treat alcohol dependency. Several studies have demonstrated its efficacy in nearly doubling rates of continuous sobriety, increasing treatment program retention rates, and decreasing the number of days of drinking in patients who were unable to maintain continuous sobriety (Garbutt *et al.*, 1999; Schaffer, 1998). Acamprosate appears to be more effective than naltrexone, and is expected to be available for use in the US soon. Its only side effect is diarrhea, which is uncommon. Acamprosate should not be used in pregnant or lactating women, or in patients with renal impairment or hepatic failure.

> Lester's liver function tests are examined, and he is started on naltrexone. He plans to return to AA, see his counselor, and follow up with his clinician within two weeks. He responds well to this treatment and after three months asks to discontinue the naltrexone. He now enjoys attending three AA meetings a week, has a sponsor, and is 'working the steps'.

Patients who are working an active program of recovery are usually eager to openly discuss their recovery with their clinicians. Frequent meeting attendance (at least one a week), contact with one's sponsor, having a 'home group', doing 'service work' and using a phone list (a list of phone numbers of the home group) have all been shown to increase a patient's chances of recovery. By asking the patient about his or her recovery, the physician can assess the 'quality' of the patient's recovery and anticipate and prevent relapses (Box 8.4) (Chappel, 1992).

Box 8.4   Alcoholics Anonymous or 12-step based questions
to assess recovery

1   How often are you going to meetings?
2   When was the last time you contacted your sponsor?
3   Do you have a home group?
4   What step are you working on?
5   When was the last time you used your phone list?

Because finding a sponsor (an active mentor with at least one year of 'recovery' in a 12-step program) can be difficult, clinicians may initially recommend a 'temporary' sponsor. Asking questions about 12-step groups is a way of assessing patient progress, as well as showing interest and support in patient recovery. Another way of demonstrating support is to recognize patient continuation in the maintenance stage. For patients choosing 12-step groups, this might mean recognition of the last day that they used drugs or alcohol, their anniversary or 'birthday'. Members of 12-step groups typically celebrate one, three, six, nine, and 12 months of recovery, and then every year thereafter.

Summary and conclusions

The patient-centered clinical method described by Stewart *et al.* (1995) embraces six components: exploring both the disease and the illness experience, understanding the whole person, finding common ground, incorporating prevention and health promotion, enhancing the patient–doctor relationship and being realistic.

Exploring both the disease and the illness experience

Dealing with a substance-abusing patient will require that Lester's clinician understands both the medical/disease model as well as Lester's ideas, expectations, feelings, and awareness of its effect on his functioning. Lester expects the visit to be related to treatment of his stomach pain and inability to relax. He also has emotions related to his wife's nagging. She will have another set of beliefs, expectations and feelings. Initially, his clinician will be unaware of these issues and will have the enormous task of addressing his stomach pain while the issues of stress and alcohol abuse are being raised.

Understanding the whole person

Understanding the whole person is essential to understanding the patient's experience. Lester's clinician will need to attend to any information that will help lead to appreciation of background issues that influenced Lester.

Finding common ground

Lester and his clinician have different perceptions of his alcohol use. How will his clinician negotiate goals and a treatment plan related to Lester's alcohol use and his health? What about his wife's expectations of the visit? Can a plan be negotiated that will address all concerns?

Incorporating prevention and health promotion

Lester comes in to address a specific concern, stomach pain. However, his clinician will need to address his total health.

Enhancing the patient–clinician relationship

This is Lester's first visit with his clinician. Power issues could emerge involving professional and gender roles of a younger, female clinician. Racial differences could also emerge as an issue of trust, along with self-awareness, transference, and countertransference issues.

Being realistic

How does a busy clinician come to grips with a 'whole person' with multiple contexts, as evidenced by our case, while dealing with the medical issues?

Lester's clinician must determine what information can be realistically gathered in this visit, a visit that includes the prospect of having to address transportation for a driving-impaired patient, and what should be left to future encounters while stewarding time and financial resources.

References

Adams SL and Waskel SA (1991) Late onset of alcoholism among older midwestern men in treatment. *Psychol Rep.* **68**: 432–4.

Addiction Research Foundation/Canadian Centre on Substance Abuse (1994) Moderate drinking and health: a joint policy statement based on the International Symposium on Moderate Drinking and Health. *CMAJ.* **151**(suppl.): 13–16.

Agnostinelli G, Brown JM and Miller WR (1995) Effects of normative feedback on consumption among heavy drinking. *J Drug Educ.* **25**(1): 31–40.

Alcoholics Anonymous (1976) *Alcoholics Anonymous: the stories of how many thousands of men and women have recovered from alcoholism* (3e). Alcoholics Anonymous World Services Inc, New York.

Allen JP, Maisto SA and Connors GJ (1995) Self-report screening tests for alcohol problems in primary care. *Arch Intern Med.* **155**: 1726–30.

Allen JP, Litten RC, Fertig JB and Babor T (1997) A review of research on the Alcohol Use Disorder Identification Test (AUDIT). *Alcohol Clin Exp Res.* **21**: 613–19.

Alvarado M and Seale D (1997) *Prevalencia de los Problemas Relacionados con Alcohol entre los Indigenas Yukpa de la Sierra de Perija* [The prevalence of problems related to alcohol among the Yukpa indigenous people of the Perija Mountains]. U.E. Colegio Bellas Artes, Maracaibo, Venezuela.

American Medical Association Committee on Alcoholism (1956) Hospitalization of patients with alcoholism (reports of officers). *JAMA.* **162**: 720.

Amodei N, Williams JF, Seale JP and Alvarado ML (1996) Gender differences in medical presentation and detection of patients with a history of alcohol abuse or dependence. *J Addict Dis.* **15**(1): 19–31.

Anderson P, Dremona A, Paton A, Thurner C and Wallace P (1993) The risk of alcohol. *Addiction.* **88**(1): 1493–508.

Andre JM (1979) *The Epidemiology of Alcoholism among American Indians and Natives.* Indian Health Service, Albuquerque, NM.

Anton RF and Moak DH (1994) Carbohydrate-deficient transferrin and gamma-glutamyl-transferase as markers of heavy alcohol consumption: gender differences. *Alcohol Clin Exp Res.* **18**(3): 747–54.

ASAM, PPC-2R (2001) *Patient Placement Criteria for the Treatment of Substance-Related Disorders* (rev 2e). American Society of Addiction Medicine Inc, Chevy Chase, MD.

Ashley MJ, Olin JS, le Riche WH *et al.* (1977) Morbidity in alcoholics: evidence for accelerated development of physical disease in women. *Arch Intern Med.* **137**(7): 883–7.

Ashley MJ, Ferrence R, Room R *et al.* (1997) Moderate drinking and health: implications of recent evidence. *Can Fam Physician.* **43**: 687–94.

Atkinson RM (1988) Alcoholism in the elderly population. *Mayo Clin Proc.* **63**(8): 825–9.

Babor TF and Grant M (1989) From clinical research to secondary prevention: international collaboration in the development of the Alcohol Use Disorders Identification Test (AUDIT). *Alcohol Health Res World.* **13**(4): 371–4.

Babor TF, de la Fuente JR, Saunders J and Grant H (1992) *AUDIT: the Alcohol Use Disorders Identification Test: guidelines for use in primary healthcare.* World Health Organization, Geneva, Switzerland.

Balint M (2000) *The Doctor, his Patient, and the Illness* (2e). Churchill Livingstone, Edinburgh, UK.

Bandura A (1977) Self-efficacy: toward a unifying theory of behavioral change. *Psychol Rev.* **84**(2): 191–215.

Barnes G, Farrell M and Banerjee S (1995) Family influences on alcohol abuse and other problem behaviors among black and white adolescents in a general population sample. In: G Boyd, J Howard and R Zucker (eds) *Alcohol Problems among Adolescents: current directions in prevention research.* Erlbaum Associates, Hillsdale, NJ.

Barry KL and Fleming MF (1993) Alcohol Use Disorders Identification Test (AUDIT) and the SMAST-13: predictive validity in a rural primary care sample. *Alcohol Alcohol.* **28**(1): 33–42.

Beck A (1976) *Cognitive Therapy and Emotional Disorders.* International Universities Press, New York.

Beck A, Wright FD, Newman CF and Liese BS (1993) *Cognitive Therapy of Substance Abuse.* The Guilford Press, New York.

Begleiter H, Porjesz B, Bihari B and Kissin B (1984) Event-related brain potentials in boys at risk for alcoholism. *Science.* **225**: 1493–6.

Beltrame T and McQueen D (1979) Urban and rural Indian drinking patterns: the special case of the Lumbee. *Int J Addict.* **14**(4): 533–48.

Benjamin D, Grant E and Pohorecky LA (1993) Naltrexone reverses ethanol-induced dopamine release in the nucleus accumbens in awake, freely moving rats. *Brain Res.* **621**: 137–40.

Bepko C (ed.) (1991) *Feminism and Addiction.* Haworth Press, New York.

Berenson D (1976) Alcohol and the family system. In: P Guerin (ed.) *Family Therapy: theory and practice.* Gardner Press, New York.

Berenstein M and Mahoney JJ (1989) Management perspectives on alcoholism: the employers' stake in alcoholism treatment. *Occup Med State Art Rev.* **4**(2): 223–32.

Beresford TP, Blow FC, Hill E, Singer K and Lucey MR (1990) Comparison of CAGE questionnaire and computer-assisted laboratory profiles in screening for covert alcoholism. *Lancet.* **336**: 482–5.

Bien TH, Miller WR and Tongan JS (1993) Brief intervention for alcohol problems: a review. *Addiction.* **88**: 315–36.

Bissell L and Skorina JK (1987) One hundred alcoholic women in medicine: an interview study. *JAMA.* **257**(21): 2939–44.

Black C (1981) Innocent bystanders at risk: the children of alcoholics. *Alcohol Clin Exp Res.* **5**: 22–5.

Blane HT and Leonard KE (1987) *Psychological Theories of Drinking and Alcoholism.* Guilford Press, New York.

Blondell RD, Graham AV and Davis AK (2000) Substance abuse. In: JW Saultz (ed.) *Textbook of Family Medicine: defining and examining the discipline.* McGraw-Hill, New York.

Blume SB (1986) Women and alcohol: a review. *J Med Assoc.* **256**(11): 1467–70.

Bongar BM (1991) *The Suicidal Patient: clinical and legal standards of care.* American Psychological Association, Washington, DC.

Booz-Allen and Hamilton Inc (1974*) An Assessment of the Needs of and Resources for Children of Alcoholic Parents.* US Department of Commerce Report PB-241–119 prepared for National Institute on Alcohol Abuse and Alcoholism, Rockville, MD.

Botelho R (1992) A negotiation model for the doctor-patient relationship. *Fam Pract.* **9**: 210–18.

Botelho R and Novak S (1993) Dealing with substance misuse, abuse, and dependency. In: RD Blondell (ed.) *Primary Care: clinics in office practice: substance abuse.* W. B. Saunders Company, Philadelphia, PA.

Bourke JG (1894) Distillation by early American Indians. *Am Anthropol.* **7**: 297–9.

Bradley KA (1994) The primary care practitioners role in the prevention and management of alcohol problems. *Alcohol Health Res World.* **18**: 97–104.

Bradley KA, Boyd-Wickizer B, Powell SH and Burman ML (1998) Alcohol screening questionnaires in women: a critical review. *JAMA.* **280**(2): 166–71.

Brehm JW (1966) *A Theory of Psychological Reactance.* Academic Press, New York.

Brennan PL and Moos RH (1991) Functioning, life context, and help seeking among late-onset problem drinkers: comparisons with non-problem and early-onset problem drinkers, *Br J Addict.* **86**: 1139–50.

British Medical Association (1995) *Alcohol: guidelines on sensible drinking.* British Medical Association, London.

Brody H (1992) *The Healer's Power.* Yale University Press, New Haven, CT.

Brown F and Tooley J (1989) Alcoholism in the Black community. In: GW Lawson and AW Lawson (eds) *Alcoholism and Substance Abuse in Special Populations.* Aspen, Gaithersburg, MD.

Brown JB and Weston WW (1995) The second component: understanding the whole person. In: M Stewart, JB Brown, WW Weston *et al.* (eds) *Patient-Centered Medicine: transforming the clinical method.* Sage Publications Inc, Thousand Oaks, CA.

Brown JB, Weston WW and Stewart M (1995) The first component: exploring both the disease and the illness perspective. In: M Stewart, J Brown, W Weston *et al.* (eds) *Patient-Centered Medicine: transforming the clinical method.* Sage Publications Inc, Thousand Oaks, CA.

Brown LM, Hoover RN, Greenberg RS *et al.* (1994) Are racial differences in squamous cell esophageal cancer explained by alcohol and tobacco use? *J Nat Cancer Inst.* **86**(17): 1340–5.

Brown LS Jr (1993) Alcohol abuse prevention in African American communities. *J Nat Med Assoc.* **85**: 665–73.

Brown RL, Leonard T, Saunders LA and Papasouliotis O (1997) A two-item screening test for alcohol and other drug problems. *J Fam Pract.* **44**(2): 151–60.

Brown S (1985) *Treating the Alcoholic: a developmental model of recovery.* Wiley, New York.

Brown S (1995) Introduction: a developmental model of alcoholism and recovery. In: S Brown and ID Yalom (eds) *Treating Alcoholism.* Jossey-Bass, San Francisco.

Buchsbaum DG, Buchanan RG, Poses RM, Schnoll SH and Lawton MJ (1992) Physician detection of drinking problems in patients attending a general medicine practice. *J Gen Intern Med.* **7**(5): 517–21.

Bulfinch T (1998) *Mythology.* Modern Library, New York.

Burge SK and Schneider FD (1999) Alcohol-related problems: recognition and intervention. *Am Fam Physician.* **15**(2): 361–70.

Burnam MA (1989) Prevalence of alcohol abuse and dependence among Mexican Americans and non-Hispanic whites in the community. In: D Spiegler, D Tate, S Aitken *et al.* (eds) *Alcohol Use Among US Ethnic Minorities.* NIAAA Research Monograph No 18. US Government Printing Office, Washington, DC.

Burns M, Daily JM and Moskowitz H (1974) *Drinking Practices and Problems of Urban American Indians in Los Angeles.* Planning Analysis and Research Institute, Santa Monica, CA.

Bush B, Shaw S, Cleary P, Delbanco TL and Aronson MD (1987) Screening for alcohol abuse using the CAGE questionnaire. *Am J Med.* **82**(2): 231–5.

Caetano R (1989) Drinking patterns and alcohol problems in a national sample of US Hispanics. In: D Spiegler, D Tate, S Aitken *et al.* (eds) *Alcohol Use Among US Ethnic Minorities.* NIAAA Research Monograph No. 18. US Government Printing Office, Washington, DC.

Caetano R (1997) Prevalence, incidence and stability of drinking problems among Whites, Blacks and Hispanics: 1984–92. *J Stud Alcohol.* **58**(6): 565–72.

Caetano R and Clark CL (1998) Trends in alcohol-related problems among Whites, Blacks, and Hispanics: 1984–95. *Alcohol Clin Exp Res.* **22**: 534–8.

Caetano R and Kaskutas LA (1995) Changes in drinking patterns among Whites, Blacks, and Hispanics: 1984–92. *J Stud Alcohol.* **56**(5): 558–65.

Caetano R and Medina Mora ME (1988) Acculturation and drinking among people of Mexican descent in Mexico and the US. *J Stud Alcohol.* **49**(5): 462–71.

Calnan M (1988) Examining the general practitioner's role in health education: a critical review. *Fam Pract.* **5**(3): 217–23.

Carmichael LP (1985) A different way of doctoring. *Fam Med.* **17**(5): 185–7.

Casswell S, Zhang JF and Wylie A (1993) The importance of amount and location of drinking for the experience of alcohol-related problems. *Addiction.* **88**: 1527–34.

Castaneda C (1974). *Teachings of Don Juan: Yagui way of knowledge.* Washington Square Press, New York.

Castaneda C (1972) *Separate Reality: further conversations with Don Juan.* Washington Square Press, New York.

Castaneda C (1987) *Power of Silence: further lessons of Don Juan.* Simon and Schuster, New York.

Chan AW, Pristach EA, Welte JW and Russell M (1993) Use of the TWEAK test: screening for alcoholism/heavy drinking in three populations. *Alcohol Clin Exp Res.* **17**(6): 1188–92.

Chan AW, Pristach EA and Welte JW (1994) Detection of alcoholism in three populations by the brief-MAST. *Alcohol Clin Exp Res.* **18**: 695–701.

Chappel JN (1992) Effective use of AA and NA in treating patients. *Psychiatr Ann.* **22**: 409–19.

Chappel JN and Lewis DC (1997) Medical education: the acquisition of knowledge, attitudes and skills. In: Lowinson JH, Ruiz P, Millman RB *et al.* (eds) *Substance Abuse: a comprehensive textbook* (3e).Williams & Wilkins, Baltimore, MD.

Chavez GF, Cordero JF and Becerra JE (1988) Leading major congenital malformations among minority groups in the US. *Morb Mortal Wkly Rep.* **37**: 17–24.

Cheever S (1999) *Note Found in a Bottle: my life as a drinker.* Simon & Schuster, New York.

Cloninger RC, Bohman M and Sigvardsson S (1981) Inheritance of alcohol abuse cross-fostering analysis of adopted men. *Arch Gen Psychiatry.* **38**: 861–8.

Cochran JK (1992) Effects of religiosity on adolescent self-reported frequency of drug and alcohol use. *J Drug Issues.* **22**(1): 91–104.

Cochran JK and Akers RL (1989) Beyond hellfire: an exploration of the variable effects of religiosity on adolescent marijuana and alcohol use. *J Res Crime Delinqu.* **26**(3): 198–225.

Coombs RH (1997) *Drug-Impaired Professionals.* Harvard University Press, Cambridge, MA.

Crabbe JC, Phillips TJ, Feller DJ *et al.* (1996) Elevated alcohol consumption in null mutant mice lacking 5-HT$_{1B}$ serotonin receptors. *Nat Genet.* **14**(1): 98–101.

Crouch MA and Roberts L (1987) *The Family in Medical Practice: a family systems primer.* Springer-Verlag, New York.

Curley RT (1967) Drinking patterns of the Mescalero Apache. *Q J Stud Alcohol.* **28**: 116–31.

Dawson DA and Archer LD (1992) Gender differences in alcohol consumption: effects of measurement. *Br J Addict.* **87**(1): 119–23.

Dawson DA and Archer LD (1993) Relative frequency of heavy drinking and the risk of alcohol dependence. *Addict.* **88**: 1509–18.

Denning P (2000) Harm reduction psychotherapy makes clinical intervention more effective. *Nat Psychol: Addictions.* **9**(4): 4-B.

Denning P (2000) Harm reduction: a primer. *Nat Psychol: Addictions.* **9**(4): 4-B–5-B.

Deykin EY, Boda SL and Zeena TH (1992) Depressive illness among chemically dependent adolescents. *Am J Psychiatry.* **149**(10): 1341–7.

DiClemente CC and Prochaska J (1998) Toward a comprehensive, transtheoretical model of change: stages of change and addictive behaviors. In: W Miller and N Heather (eds) *Treating Addictive Behaviors.* Plenum, New York.

Donovan DM (1998) Continuing care. In: W Miller and N Heather (eds) *Treating Addictive Behaviors.* Plenum, New York.

Egeland GM, Perham-Hester KA, Gessner BD *et al.* (1998) Fetal alcohol syndrome in Alaska, 1977–92: an administrative prevalence derived from multiple data sources. *Am J Public Health.* **88**(5): 781–6.

Ellis A, McInerney JF, DiGuiseppe R and Yeager RJ (1988) *Rational-Emotive Therapy with Alcohol and Substance Abusers.* Pergamon Press, Elmsford, New York.

Elster AB and Kunznets NJ (eds) (1994) *AMA Guidelines for Adolescent Preventive Services (GAPS).* Williams & Wilkins, Baltimore, MD.

Epstein R (1999) Mindful practice. *JAMA.* **282**: 833–9.

Epstein R, Campbell T, Choen-Cole S, McWhinney L and Smilkstein G (1983) Perspectives on patient–doctor communication. *J Fam Pract.* **37**(4): 377–88.

Erikson EH (1963) *Childhood and Society.* W. W. Norton & Co, New York.

Ewing JA (1984) Detecting alcoholism: the CAGE questionnaire. *JAMA.* **252**(14): 1905–7.

Fink A, Hays RD, Moore AA and Beck JC (1996) Alcohol-related problems in older persons: determinants, consequences and screening. *Arch Intern Med.* **156**: 1150–6.

Fisher R and Ury W (1983) *Getting to Yes: negotiating agreement without giving in.* Penguin, New York.

Fisher S (1995) *Nursing Wounds: nurse practitioners, doctors, women patients, and the negotiation of meaning.* Rutgers University Press, New Brunswick, NJ.

Fleming M (1991) *Detoxification.* Paper presented at the meeting of The Society of Teachers of Family Medicine on the Project SAEFP Syllabus, Kansas City, MO.

Fleming M (1993) Screening and brief intervention for alcohol disorders. *J Fam Pract.* **37**(3): 231–4.

Fleming M and Murray M (1997) *An International Medical Education Model for the Prevention and Treatment of Alcohol Use Disorders.* National Institute on Alcohol Abuse and Alcoholism, Bethesda, MD.

Fleming M and Barry KL (1991) A three-sample test of an alcohol screening questionnaire. *Alcohol Alcohol.* **26**: 81–91.

Fleming M, Barry, KL, Manwell LB, Johnson K and London R (1997) Brief physician advice for problem drinkers: a randomized controlled trial in community-based primary care practices. *JAMA.* **277**: 1039–45.

Fleming M, Manwell LB, Barry KL and Johnson K (1998) At-risk drinking in an HMO primary care sample: prevalence and health policy implications. *Am J Public Health.* **88**: 90–3.

Floren AE (1994) Urine drug screening and the family physician. *Am Fam Physician.* **49**(6): 1441–7.

Frezza M, di Podava C, Pozzato G *et al.* (1990) High blood alcohol levels in women: the role of decreased gastric dehydrogenase activity and first-pass metabolism. *N Engl J Med.* **322**(2): 95–9.

Fuller RK, Branchney L, Brightwell DR *et al.* (1986) Disulfiram treatment of alcoholism: a veterans administration cooperative study. *JAMA.* **256**(11): 1449–55.

Garbutt JC, West SL, Carey TS, Lohr KN and Crews FT (1999) Pharmacological treatment of alcohol dependence: a review of the evidence. *JAMA.* **281**(14): 1318–25.

Gardner EL (1997) Brain reward mechanisms. In: JH Lowinson *et al.* (eds) *Substance Abuse.* Williams & Wilkins, Baltimore, MD.

George FR (1987) Genetic and environmental factors in ethanol self-administration. *Pharmacol Biochem Behav.* **27**: 379–84.

Gerber GJ and Stretch R (1975) Drug-induced reinstatement of extinguished self-administration behavior in monkeys. *Pharmacol Biochem Behav.* **3**: 1055–61.

Gerson R (1995) The family lifecycle: phases, stages and crises. In: RH Mikesell, DD Lusterman and SH McDaniel (eds) *Integrating Family Therapy: handbook of family psychology and systems theory.* American Psychological Association, Washington DC.

Gerson R and Shellenberger S (2001) *The Genogram-Maker Millennium.* GenoWare Inc, Macon, GA.

Gibbon E (1932) *The Decline and Fall of the Roman Empire.* Modern Library, New York.

Gilbert MJ (1985) Mexican Americans in California: intercultural variations in attitudes and behavior related to alcohol. In: LA Bennett and GM Ames (eds) *The American Experience with Alcohol.* Plenum, New York.

Gilbert MJ (1989) Alcohol-related practices, problems, and norms among Mexican Americans: an overview. In: D Spiegler, D Tate, S Aitken *et al.* (eds) *Alcohol Use Among US Ethnic Minorities.* Research Monograph No. 18. National Institute on Alcohol Abuse and Alcoholism, Rockville, MD.

Gilbert MJ and Cervantes RC (1986) Patterns and practices of alcohol use among Mexican-Americans: a comprehensive review. *Hisp J Behav Sci.* **8**(1): 1–60.

Gillis AJ (1993) Determinants of a health-promoting lifestyle: an integrative review. *J Adv Nurs.* **18**: 345–53.

Gomberg ES (1993) Recent developments in alcoholism: gender issues. *Recent Dev Alcohol.* **11**: 95–107.

Gomberg ES (1998) Social predictions of women's alcohol and drug use: implications for prevention and treatment. In: AW Graham and TK Schultz (eds) *Principles of Addiction* (2e). American Society of Addiction Medicine Inc, Chevy Chase, MD.

Goodwin D (1985) Alcoholism and genetics. *Arch Gen Psychiatry.* **42**: 171–4.

Goodwin D (1990) *Alcohol and the Writer.* Penguin, New York.

Goodwin D, Schulsinger F, Hermansen L, Guze SB and Winokur G (1973) Alcohol problems in adoptees raised apart from alcoholic biological parents. *Arch Gen Psychiatry.* **28**: 238–43.

Goodwin FK (1990) Co-morbidity of mental disorders with alcohol and other drug abuse: results from the Epidemiologic Catchment Area (ECA) study. *JAMA.* **264**(19): 2511–18.

Gordon T (1970) *PET: Parent Effectiveness Training.* Van Rees Press, New York.

Graham JW, Johnson CA, Hansen WB, Flay BR and Gee M (1990) Drug use prevention programs, gender and ethnicity: evaluation of three seventh-grade project SMART cohorts. *Prev Med.* **19**(3): 305–13.

Graham K (1986) Identifying and measuring alcohol abuse among the elderly: serious problems with existing instrumentation. *J Stud Alcohol.* **47**: 322–6.

Grant B (1997a) *The Relationship Between Age of First Drink and the Risk of Lifetime Alcohol Abuse or Dependence.* Analysis of national survey data prepared for the Director. National Institute on Alcohol Abuse and Alcoholism, Rockville, MD.

Grant B (1997b) Prevalence and correlates of alcohol use and DSM IV alcohol dependence in the US: results of the National Longitudinal Epidemiologic Alcohol Survey. *J Stud Alcohol.* **58**(5): 464–73.

Grant B, Harford TC, Dawson DA *et al.* (1994) Prevalence of DSM IV alcohol abuse and dependence: US 1992. *Alcohol Health Res World.* **18**(3): 243–8.

Group for the Advancement of Psychiatry (1996) *Alcoholism in the US: racial and ethnic considerations.* American Psychiatric Press Inc, Washington, DC.

Grove WM, Eckert ED, Heston L *et al.* (1990) Heritability of substance abuse and anti-social behavior: a study of monozygotic twins reared apart. *Biol Psychiatry.* **27**(12): 1293–304.

Haines M and Spear SF (1996) Changing the perception of the norm: a strategy to decrease binge drinking among college students. *J Am Coll Health.* **45**(3): 134–40.

Haley J (1977) Toward a theory of pathological systems. In: P Watzlawick and J Weakland (eds) *The Interactional View.* Norton, New York.

Hansen WB, Graham JW, Wolkenstein B *et al.* (1988) Differential impact of three alcohol prevention curricula on hypothesized mediating variables. *J Drug Educ.* **18**(2): 143–53.

Harburg E, DiFranceisco W and Webster DW (1990) A familial transmission of alcohol use: imitation of and aversion to parent drinking (1960) by adult offspring (1977). Tecumseh, Michigan. *J Stud Alcohol.* **51**(3): 245–56.

Harford TC and Grant BF (1994) Prevalence and population validity of DCM-III-R alcohol abuse and dependence: the 1989 National Longitudinal Survey on Youth. *J Subst Abuse.* **6**(1): 37–44.

Heath DB (1989) American Indians and alcohol: epidemiological and sociocultural relevance. In: D Spiegler, D Tate, S Aitken *et al.* (eds) *Alcohol Use Among US Ethnic Minorities.* Research Monograph No. 18. National Institute on Alcohol Abuse and Alcoholism, Rockville, MD.

Hecht M (1973) Children of alcoholics are children at risk. *Am J Nurs.* **73**(10): 1764–7.

Helzer JE, Burnam A and McEvory LT (1991) Alcohol abuse and dependence. In: LN Robins and DA Regier (eds) *Psychiatric Disorders in America.* Free Press, New York.

Henson LP (1998) Variables influencing adolescent experiences with alcohol and the church. *Diss Abstr Int.* **58**(8): 4523-B.

Herd D (1990) Subgroup differences in drinking patterns among Black and White men: results from a national survey. *J Stud Alcohol.* **51**: 221–32.

Herd D (1994) Predicting drinking problems among Black and White men: results from a national survey. *J Stud Alcohol.* **55**(1): 61–71.

Hingson R and Howland J (1989) Alcohol, injury and legal controls: some complex interactions. *Law Med Health Care.* **17**(1): 58–68.

Hird S, Khuri ET, Dusenberry L and Millman RB (1997) Adolescents. In: JH Lowinsohn, P Ruiz, RB Millman *et al.* (eds) *Substance Abuse: a comprehensive textbook* (3e). Williams & Wilkins, Baltimore, MD.

Holder HD (1987) Alcoholism treatment and potential healthcare costs savings. *Med Care.* **25**(1): 52–71.

Homer (1963) *The Odyssey* (trans. Fitzgerald R). Anchor Books, Garden City, NY.

Horvath AT (2000) Alcoholism: 12-step isn't for everyone. *Nat. Psychol: Addictions.* **9**(4): 1B–2B.

Howard J, Boyd G and Zucker R (1995) An overview of issues. In: G Boyd, J Howard and R Zucker (eds) *Alcohol Problems Among Adolescents: current directions in prevention research.* Erlbaum Associates, Hillsdale, NJ.

Hrubec Z and Omenn GS (1991) Evidence of genetic predisposition to alcoholic cirrhosis and psychosis: twin concordances for alcoholism and its biological end points by zygosity among male veterans. *Alcohol Clin Exp Res.* **5**: 207–15.

Hudak J, Krestan J and Bepko C (1998) Alcohol problems and the family life cycle. In: B Carter and M McGoldrick (eds) *The Expanded Family Life Cycle: individual, family and social perspectives* (3e). Allyn & Bacon, Boston, MA.

Hudson HL (1986) How and why Alcoholics Anonymous works for Blacks. *Alcohol Treat Q.* **2**(3–4): 11–29.

Hughes TL, Day LE, Marcantonio RJ and Torpy E (1997) Gender differences in alcohol and other drug use among young adults. *Subst Use Misuse.* **32**(3): 317–42.

Hunt RD, Finlayson RE, Morse RM and Davis LJ (1988) Alcoholism in elderly persons: medical aspects and prognosis of 216 inpatients. *Mayo Clin Proc.* **63**(8): 753–60.

Imber-Black E, Roberts J and Whiting R (eds) (1988) *Rituals in Families and Family Therapy.* Norton, New York.

Indian Health Service (1990) *Trends in Indian Health 1990.* Office of Planning, Evaluation and Legislation, Division of Program Statistics, US Indian Health Service, Rockville, MD.

Institute of Medicine, Division of Mental Health and Behavioral Medicine (1990) *Broadening the Base of Treatment for Alcohol Problems.* National Academy Press, Washington, DC.

Jacob T (1992) Family studies of alcoholism. *J Fam Psychol.* **5**: 319–38.

Jacob T and Krahn G (1988) Marital interactions of alcoholic couples: comparison with depressed and non-distressed couples. *J Consult Clin Psychol.* **56**(1): 73–9.

Jacob T and Leonard K (1994) Family and peer influences in the development of adolescent alcohol abuse. In: R Zucker, G Boyd and J Howard (eds) *The Development of Alcohol Problems: exploring the bio-psycho-social matrix of risk.* National Institute on Alcohol Abuse and Alcoholism, Rockville, MD.

Jacobs J and Wolin SJ (1991) *Resilient children growing up in alcoholic families.* Paper presented at the National Consensus Symposium on Children of Alcoholics and Co-Dependence, Warrenton, VA.

JAMA 100 Years Ago (1994) The disease of inebriety. *JAMA.* **Dec. 28.**

Jellinek EM (1946) Phases in the drinking history of alcoholics: analysis of a survey conducted by the official organ of Alcoholics Anonymous. *Q J Stud Alcohol.* **7**: 1–88.

Jellinek EM (1952) Phases of alcohol addiction. *Q J Stud Alcohol.* **13**: 673–84.

Jernigan D (1991) Alcohol and head trauma. *J Head Traum Rehab.* **62**: 48–59.

Jernigan D, Mosher J and Reed D (1989) Alcohol-related problems and public hospitals: defining a new role in prevention. *J Pub Health Policy.* **10**(3): 324–52.

Jessor R (1983) *Adolescent Problem Drinking: psychosocial aspects and developmental outcomes.* Proceedings of the NIAAA-WHO Collaborating Center Designation Meeting and Alcohol Research Seminar, 31 October–2 November, Washington DC.

Johnson S (1978) *Cirrhosis Mortality Among American Indian Women: rates and ratios, 1975. Working Paper 6.* Alcohol Epidemiologic Data System, Rockville, MD.

Johnston LD, O'Malley PM and Bachman JG (1993) *National Survey Results on Drug Use from the Monitoring the Future Study, 1975–92.* National Institute on Drug Abuse Publication, US Government Printing Office, Washington, DC.

Johnston LD, O'Malley PM and Bachman JG (1996) *National Survey Results on Drug Use from the Monitoring the Future Study, 1975–94: College students and young adults.* US Department of Health and Human Services, Public Health Service, National Institutes of Health, National Institute on Drug Abuse, Rockville, MD.

Johnston LD, O'Malley PM and Bachman JG (1998) *National Survey Results on Drug Use from the Monitoring the Future Study, 1975–97: Secondary school students.* US Department of Health and Human Services, Public Health Service, National Institutes of Health, National Institute on Drug Abuse, Rockville, MD.

Jones MC (1971) Personality antecedents and correlates of drinking patterns in women. *J Consult Clin Psychol.* **36**: 61–9.

Jorenby DE (1997) *Effects of Nicotine on the Central Nervous System: hospital practice: a special report.* McGraw Hill, New York.

Kahan M (1996) Identifying and managing problem drinkers. *Can Fam Physician.* **42**: 661–71.

Kaij L (1960) *Studies on the Etiology and Sequels of Abuse of Alcohol.* University of Lund, Sweden.

Kaprio J, Koskenvuo M, Langinvainio H *et al.* (1987) Genetic influences on use and abuse of alcohol: a study of 5638 adult Finnish twin brothers. *Alcoholism.* **11**(4): 349–56.

Kaufman E and Pattison M (1990) Differential methods of family therapy in the treatment of alcoholism. In: D Ward (ed.) *Alcoholism: introduction to theory and treatment* (3e). Kendall/Hunt, Dubuque, IA.

Kendler K, Heath A, Neale M, Kessler R and Eaves L (1992) A population-based twin study of alcoholism in women. *JAMA.* **268**: 1877–82.

Kendler K, Bulik CM, Silberg J *et al.* (2000) Childhood sexual abuse and adult psychiatric and substance use disorders in women: an epidemiological and co-twin analysis. *Arch Gen Psychiatry.* **57**(10): 953–9.

Khantzian EJ and Mack JE (1989) Alcoholics Anonymous and contemporary psychodynamic theory. In: M Galanter (ed.) *Recent Developments in Alcoholism.* Plenum, New York.

Klitzner M, Vegega ME and Gruenwald P (1988) An empirical examination of the assumptions underlying youth drinking/driving prevention programs. *Eval Program Plan.* **11**: 219–35.

Knapp C (1997) *Drinking: a love story.* Bantam Doubleday Dell Publishing Group, New York.

Knight JR, Shrier LA, Bravender TD *et al.* (1999) A new brief screen for adolescent substance abuse. *Arch Pediatr Adolesc Med.* **153**(6): 591–6.

Knox DH (1986) Spirituality: a tool in the assessment and treatment of Black alcoholics and their families. *Alcohol Treat Q.* **2**(3–4): 11–29.

Komro KA, Perry CL, Murray DM *et al.* (1996). Peer-planned social activities for preventing alcohol use among young adolescents. *J Sch Health.* **66**: 328–34.

Krestan J and Bepko C (1989) Alcohol problems and the family lifecycle. In: B Carter and M McGoldrick (eds) *The Changing Family Lifecycle* (2e). Allyn and Bacon, Needhan Heights, MA.

Krystal H (1979) Alexithymia psychotherapy. *Am J Psychother.* **33**(01): 17–31.

Kutter CJ and McDermott DS (1997) Role of the church in adolescent drug education. *J Drug Educ.* **27**(3): 293–305.

Kutz DL (1996) Subjective culture and the workplace: comparing Hispanic and mainstream naval recruits. *Mil Med.* **161**(2): 78–83.

Lamarine RJ (1988) Alcohol abuse among Native Americans. *J Community Health.* **13**(3): 143–55.

Lang F and McCord RS (1999) Agenda setting in the patient–physician relationship (letter). *JAMA.* **282**(10): 942.

Lang F, Floyd M and Beine K (2000) Clues to patients' explanations and concerns about their illnesses: a call for active listening. *Arch Fam Med.* **9**: 222–7.

Lang F, Floyd M, Beine K *et al.* (1998) *Reaching Common Ground: core interview skills of a patient-centered interview*. Department of Family Medicine, East Tennessee State University, Johnson City, TN.

Lawson A (1990) Group therapy for adult children of alcoholics. In: D Ward (ed.) *Alcoholism: introduction to theory and treatment* (3e). Kendall/Hunt, Dubuque, IA.

Leeds J and Morgenstern J (1996) Psychoanalytic theories in substance abuse. In: F Rotgers, DS Keller and J Morgenstern (eds) *Treating Substance Abuse: theory and technique*. Guilford Press, New York.

Lemert EM (1982) Drinking among American Indians. In: EL Gomberg, HR White and JA Carpenter (eds) *Alcohol, Science and Society Revisited*. University of Michigan Press, Ann Arbor, MI.

Leonard K and Blane HT (1999) *Psychological Theories of Drinking and Alcoholism* (2e). Guilford Publications, New York.

Leonard K and Jacob T (1988) Alcohol, alcoholism and family violence. In: VB Van Hasselt, RL Morrison, S Bellack *et al.* (eds) *Handbook of Family Violence*. Plenum, New York.

Leshner A (2000) *Principles of Drug Abuse Treatment: a research-based guide*. The National Institute on Drug Abuse, Rockville, MD.

Leung PK, Kinzie JD, Boehnlein JK and Shore JH (1993) A prospective study of the natural course of alcoholism in a Native American village. *J Stud Alcohol.* **54**: 733–8.

Levenstein JH (1984) The patient-centered general practice consultation. *S Afr Fam Pract.* **5**: 276–82.

Levin JD (1995) Psychodynamic treatment of alcohol abuse. In: JP Barber and P Crits-Cristoph (eds) *Dynamic Therapies for Psychiatric Disorders: Axis I*. Basic Books, New York.

Levy JE and Kunitz S (1974) *Indian Drinking: Navaho practices and Anglo-American theories*. Wiley, New York.

Lewis DC (1994) A disease model of addiction. In: NS Miller (ed.) *Principles of Addiction Medicine*. ASAM, Chevy Chase, MD.

Lex BW (1991) Some gender differences in alcohol and polysubstance users. *Health Psychol.* **10**(2): 121–32.

Li TK, Lumeng L and McBride WJ (1979) Progress toward a voluntary oral consumption model of alcoholism. *Drug Alcohol Depend.* **4**(1–2): 45–60.

Liberto JG, Oslin DW and Ruskin PE (1992) Alcoholism in older persons: a review of the literature. *Hosp Community Psychiatry.* **43**(10): 975–84.

Liebschutz JM, Mulvey KP and Samet JH (1997) Victimization among substance-abusing women. *Arch Intern Med.* **157**: 1093–7.

Little P, Everitt H, Williamson I *et al.* (2001) Preferences of patients for patient-centred approach to consultation in primary care: observational study. *BMJ.* **322**(7284): 468–72.

Mail PD and Johnson S (1993) Boozing, sniffing, and toking: an overview of the past, present and future of substance use by American Indians. *Am Indian Alsk Native Ment Health Res.* **5**(2): 1–33.

Manson SM, Shore JH, Baron AE, Ackerson L and Neligh G (1992) Alcohol abuse and dependence among American Indians. In: JE Helzer and JG Canino (eds) *Alcoholism in North America, Europe, and Asia.* Oxford University Press, New York.

Margolis RD and Zweben JE (1998) *Treating Patients with Alcohol and Other Drug Problems: an integrated approach.* American Psychological Association, Washington, DC.

Marks G, Graham JW and Hansen WB (1992) Social projection and social conformity in adolescent alcohol use: a longitudinal analysis. *Perspect Soc Psychol Bull.* **18**(1): 96–101.

Marlatt GA and VandenBos GR (1997) *Addictive Behaviors: readings on etiology, prevention and treatment.* American Psychological Association, Washington, DC.

Maslow AH (1968) *Toward a Psychology of Being.* Van Nostrand Reinhold, Princeton, NJ.

Mason BJ, Salvato FR, Williams LD, Ritvo EC and Cutler RB (1999) A double-blind, placebo-controlled study of oral Nalmefene for alcohol dependence. *Arch Gen Psychiatry.* **56**(8): 719–24.

Mason RD, Mail PD, Palmer I and Zephier RL (1985) *Briefing Book for the Alcoholism Program Review.* Program Branch, Indian Health Service. Albuquerque, NM.

May PA (1982) Substance abuse and American Indians: prevalence and susceptibility. *Int J Addict.* **17**(7): 1185–209.

May PA, Hymbaugh KJ, Aase JM and Samet JM (1983) Epidemiology of fetal alcohol syndrome among American Indians of the South-west. *Soc Biol.* **30**: 344–87.

Mayfield D, McLeod G and Hall P (1974) The CAGE questionnaire: validation of a new alcoholism screening instrument. *Am J Psychiatry.* **131**: 1121–3.

Mayo-Smith MF (1998) Pharmacological management of alcohol withdrawal: a meta-analysis and evidence-based practice guideline. *JAMA.* **278**(2): 144–51.

McGoldrick M, Gerson R and Shellenberger S (1999) *Genograms: assessment and intervention.* W. W. Norton, New York.

McGue M, Pickens RW and Svikis DS (1992) Sex and age effects on the inheritance of alcohol problems: a twin study. *J Abnorm Psychol.* **101**(1): 3–17.

McMenamin JP (1994) Screening for alcohol use disorder in a general practice. *NZ Med J.* **107**(972): 55–7.

McWhinney IR (1972) Beyond diagnosis: an approach to the integration of behavioral science and clinical medicine. *NEJM.* **287**: 384–7.

McWilliam CL and Freeman, TR (1995) The fourth component: incorporating prevention and health promotion. In: M Stewart, JB Brown, WW Weston *et al.* (eds) *Patient-Centered Medicine: transforming the clinical method.* Sage Publications Inc, Thousand Oaks, CA.

Medicine B (1982) New roads to coping: Siouan sobriety. In: SM Manson (ed.) *New Directions in Prevention among American Indian and Alaskan Native Communities.* Oregon Health Sciences University, Portland, OR.

Mendenhall CL, Gartside PS, Roselle GA *et al.* (1989) Longevity among ethnic groups in alcoholic liver disease. *Alcohol Alcohol.* **24**(1): 11–19.

Mercer PW and Khavari KA (1990) Are women drinking more like men?: an empirical examination of the convergence hypothesis. *Alcohol Clin Exp Res.* **14**(3): 461–6.

Mezey E, Kolman CJ, Diehl AM, Mitchell MC and Herlong HF (1988) Alcohol and dietary intake in the development of chronic pancreatitis and liver disease in alcoholism. *Am J Clin Nutr.* **48**(1): 148–51.

Midanik LT and Clark WB (1994) Demographic distribution of US drinking patterns in 1990: description and trends from 1984. *Am J Pub Health.* **84**(8): 1218–22.

Midanik LT and Clark WB (1995) Drinking-related problems in the US: description and trends, 1984–90. *J Stud Alcohol.* **56**(4): 395–402.

Midanik LT, Tam TW, Greenfield TK and Caetano R (1996) Risk functions for alcohol-related problems in a 1988 US national sample. *Addiction.* **91**(10): 1427–37.

Miller NS, Belkin BM and Gold MS (1991) Alcohol and drug dependence among the elderly: epidemiologic, diagnosis and treatment. *Compr Psychiatry.* **32**: 153–65.

Miller WR and Heather N (1998) *Treating Addictive Behaviors* (2e). Plenum, New York.

Miller WR and Rollnick S (1991) *Motivational Interviewing: preparing people to change addictive behavior.* Guilford Press, New York.

Minuchin S (1974) *Families and Family Therapy.* Harvard University Press, Cambridge, MA.

Montgomery CL (1993) *Healing Through Communication: the practice of caring.* Sage Publications Inc, Newbury Park, CA.

Moore M and Weiss S (1995) Reasons for non-drinking among Israeli adolescents of four religions. *Drug Alcohol Depend.* **38**(1): 45–50.

Moore RD and Malitz FE (1986) Underdiagnosis of alcoholism by residents in an ambulatory medical practice. *J Med Educ.* **61**(1): 46–52.

Moran M (1985) *Lost Years: confessions of a woman alcoholic.* Doubleday, Garden City, NJ.

Morrison MA (1989) *White Rabbit: a doctor's own story of addiction, survival and recovery.* Berkley Books, New York.

Morse RM and Flavin DK (1992) The definition of alcoholism. *JAMA.* **268**(8): 1012–14.

Moss FE (1979) *Drinking Attitudes and Practices in Twenty Indian Communities.* Western Region Alcoholism Training Center, University of Utah, Salt Lake City, UT.

Murphy JM, McBride WJ, Lumeng L and Li TK (1982) Regional brain levels of monoamines in alcohol-preferring and non-preferring lines of rats. *Pharmacol Biochem Behav.* **16**(1): 145–9.

Murphy JM, McBride WJ, Lumeng L and Li TK (1987) Contents of monoamines in forebrain regions of alcohol-preferring (P) and non-preferring (NP) lines of rats. *Pharmacol Biochem Behav.* **26**(2): 389–92.

Murray RM and Clifford HD (1983) Twin and adoption studies: how good is the evidence for a genetic role? In: M Galanter (ed.) *Recent Developments in Alcoholism, Vol. 1*. Plenum, New York.

Nace EP (1997) Alcoholics Anonymous. In: JH Lowinsohn, P Ruiz, RB Millman *et al.* (eds) *Substance Abuse: a comprehensive textbook* (3e). Williams & Wilkins, Baltimore, MD.

National Center for Health Statistics (1987) *Drug Abuse: ages 12 years to 74 years. Version I: Hispanic Health and Nutrition Examination Survey, 1982–84. Public Use Data Tape Documentation No. 6543*. NCHS, US Department of Health and Human Services, Public Health Services, Washington, DC.

National Center for Health Statistics (1997) *Report of Final Mortality Statistics, 1995*. Monthly Vital Statistics Report, NCHS, Hyattsville, MD.

National Institute on Alcohol Abuse and Alcoholism (1995) *The Physicians' Guide to Helping Patients with Alcohol Problems*. US Department of Health and Human Services, Public Health Service, National Institutes of Health, NIAAA, Washington, DC.

National Institute on Drug Abuse (1996) *National Pregnancy and Health Survey: drug use among women delivering livebirths: 1992*. US Department of Health and Human Services, Public Health Service, National Institutes of Health, National Institute on Drug Abuse, Division of Epidemiology and Prevention Research, NIDA, Rockville, MD.

National Institute on Drug Abuse (1998) *Drug Use Among Racial/Ethnic Minorities*. US Department of Health and Human Services, Public Health Service, National Institutes of Health, National Institute on Drug Abuse, Division of Epidemiology and Prevention Research, NIDA, Rockville, MD.

Newcomb M (1994) Family, peers, and adolescent alcohol abuse: a paradigm to study: multiple causes, mechanisms, and outcomes. In: R Zucker, G Boyd and J Howard (eds) *The Development of Alcohol Problems: exploring the bio-psycho-social matrix of risk*. National Institute on Alcohol Abuse and Alcoholism, Rockville, MD.

Nobles WW (1972) African philosophy: foundations for black psychology. In: RL Jones (ed.) *Black Psychology*. Harper & Row, New York.

Oetting E and Beauvais F (1989) Epidemiology and correlates of alcohol use among Indian adolescents living on reservations. In: D Spiegler, DA Tate, AC Aitken and C Christian (eds) *Alcohol Use among US Ethnic Minorities*. Research Monograph No. 18. National Institute on Alcohol Abuse and Alcoholism, Rockville, MD.

O'Farrell T (ed.) (1993) *Treating Alcohol Problems: marital and family interventions*. Guilford Press, New York.

O'Malley SS, Jaffe AJ, Chang G *et al.* (1992) Naltrexone and coping skills therapy for alcohol dependence: a controlled study. *Arch Gen Psychiatry*. **49**(11): 881–7.

Opler ME (1941) *An Apache Life-way*. The University of Chicago Press, Chicago, IL.

O'Sullivan C (1991) Making a difference: the relationship between childhood mentors and resiliency in adult children of alcoholics. *Fam Dynam Addict Q*. **1**(4): 46–59.

Parish DC (1997) Another indication for screening and early intervention: problem drinking. *JAMA*. **277**(13): 1079–80.

Peabody FW (1984) The care of the patient. *JAMA.* **252**: 813–18.

Perkins HW and Wechsler H (1996) Variation in perceived college drinking norms and its impact on alcohol abuse: a nationwide study. *J Drug Issues.* **26**(4): 961–74.

Perkins HW, Meilman PW, Leichliter JS, Cashin JR and Presley CA (1999) Misperceptions of the norms for the frequency of alcohol and other drug use on college campuses. *J Am Coll Health.* **47**(6): 253–8.

Peterson P, Hawkins JD, Abbott RD and Catalan RF (1995) Disentangling the effects of parental drinking, family management and parental alcohol norms on current drinking by Black and White adolescents. In: G Boyd, J Howard and R Zucker (eds) *Alcohol Problems among Adolescents: current directions in prevention research.* Erlbaum Associates, Hillsdale, NJ.

Pickens RW, Svikis DS, McGue M *et al.* (1991) Heterogeneity in the inheritance of alcoholism. *Arch Gen Psychiatry.* **48**(1): 19–28.

Pokorny AD and Kanas TE (1980) Stages in the development of alcoholism. In: WE Farr, I Karacan, AD Pokorny *et al.* (eds) *Phenomenology and Treatment of Alcoholism.* SP Medical and Scientific Books, New York.

Polednak AP (1997) Gender and acculturation in relation to alcohol use among Hispanic (Latino) adults in two areas of the northeastern United States. *Subst Use Misuse.* **32**: 1513–24.

Porter R (1997) *The Greatest Benefit of Mankind: a medical history of humanity.* Harper Collins, New York.

Prochaska JO and DiClemente CC (1983) Stages and processes of self-change in smoking: toward an integrative model of change. *J Consult Clin Psychology.* **5**: 390–5.

Prochaska J and DiClemente C (1986) *Toward a Comprehensive Model of Protocol: (TIP) Series 26.* US Department of Health and Human Services, Rockville, MD.

Prochaska JO, DiClemente CC and Norcross JC (1992) In search of how people change. *Am Psychol.* **47**: 1102–4.

Quinby PM and Graham AV (1993) Substance abuse among women. In: RD Blondell (ed.) *Primary Care Clinics in Office Practice: substance abuse. Vol. 20, No. 1.* W.B. Saunders Company, Philadelphia, PA.

Regier DA, Farmer ME, Rae DS *et al.* (1990) Co-morbidity of mental disorders with alcohol and other drug abuse: results from the Epidemiologic Catchment Area (ECA) study. *JAMA.* **264**(19): 2511–18.

Reid MC and Anderson PA (1997) Geriatric substance use disorders. *Med Clin North Am.* **81**: 999–1016.

Resnick MD, Bearman PS, Blum RW *et al.* (1997) Protecting adolescents from harm: findings from the National Longitudinal Study on Adolescent Health. *JAMA.* **278**(10): 823–32.

Rich CL, Fowler RC, Fogarty LA and Young D (1988) San Diego suicide study III: relationships between diagnoses and stressors. *Arch Gen Psychiatry.* **45**(6): 589–92.

Richards A (1989) Alcohol is a woman's issue. *Counselor.* **January/February**: 15–20.

Robin RW, Long JC, Rasmussen JK, Albaugh B and Goldman D (1998) Relationship of binge drinking to alcohol dependence, other psychiatric disorders and behavioral problems in an American Indian tribe. *Alcohol Clin Exp Res.* **22**: 518–23.

Robins LN and Murphy GE (1967) Drug use in a normal population of young Negro men. *Am J Public Health.* **57**: 1580–96.

Rollnick S, Heather N and Bell A (1992) Negotiating behaviour change in medical settings: the development of brief motivational interviewing. *J Ment Health.* **1**: 25–37.

Rollnick S, Mason P and Butler C (1999) *Health Behavior Change: a guide for practitioners.* Churchill Livingstone, Toronto.

Roman PM (1988) *Women and Alcohol Use: a review of the research literature.* US Department of Health and Human Services, Rockville, MD.

Room R, Bondy SJ and Ferris J (1995) The risk of harm to oneself from drinking. *Addiction.* **90**: 499–513.

Rosenbaum EE (1988) *The Doctor.* Ballantine Books, New York.

Rosenberg SD and Farrell MP (1976) Identity and crisis in middle-aged men. *Int J Aging Hum Dev.* **1**: 153.

Rosman AS and Lieber CS (1990) Biochemical markers of alcohol consumption. *Alcohol Health Res World.* **14**(3): 210–18.

Rotunda R, Scherer D and Imm P (1995) Family systems and alcohol misuse: research on the effects of alcoholism on family functioning and effective family interventions. *Pro Psychol Res Pract.* **26**: 95–104.

Rouse B (1989) *Drug Abuse among Racial/Ethnic Minorities: a special report.* National Institute of Drug Abuse, Rockville, MD.

Rozynko V and Ferguson LC (1978) Admission characteristics of Indian and White alcoholic patients in a rural mental hospital. *Int J Addict.* **13**: 591–604.

Rush BR (1989) The use of family medical practices by patients with drinking problems. *Can Med Assoc J.* **140**(1): 35–8.

Russell M, Martier SS, Sokol RJ *et al.* (1994) Screening for pregnancy risk-drinking. *Alcohol Clin Exp Res.* **18**(5): 1156–61.

Russell M, Martier SS, Sokol RJ *et al.* (1996) Detecting risk drinking during pregnancy: a comparison of four screening questionnaires. *Am J Public Health.* **86**(10): 1435–9.

Saitz R, Mayo-Smith MF, Roberts MS *et al.* (1994) Individualized treatment of alcohol withdrawal. *JAMA.* **272**(7): 519–23.

Satel SL, Kosten TR, Schuckit MA and Fischman MW (1993) Should protracted withdrawal from drugs be included in DSM IV? *Am J Psychiatry.* **150**: 695–704.

Saunders JB, Aasland OG, Amundsen A and Grant M (1993a) Alcohol consumption and related problems among primary health care patients: WHO collaborative project on early detection of persons with harmful alcohol consumption – Part 1. *Addiction.* **88**: 349–62.

Saunders JB, Aasland OG, Babor TF, De la Fuente JR and Grant M (1993b) Development of the Alcohol Use Disorders Identification Test (AUDIT): WHO collaborative project on early detection of persons with harmful alcohol consumption. Part II. *Addiction.* **88**: 791–804.

Schaffer A and Naranjo C (1998) Recommended drug treatment strategies for the alcoholic patient. *Drugs.* **56**(4): 571–85.

Schuckit MA (1999) New findings in the genetics of alcoholism. *JAMA.* **281**(20): 1875–6.

Schuckit MA and Gold EO (1988) A simultaneous evaluation of multiple markers of ethanol/ placebo challenges in sons of alcoholics and controls. *Arch Gen Psychiatry.* **45**(3): 211–16.

Schuckit MA and Smith TL (1996) An 8-year follow-up of 450 sons of alcoholic and control subjects. *Arch Gen Psychiatry.* **53**: 202–10.

Schuckit MA, Mazzanti C, Smith T *et al.* (1999) Selective genotyping for the role of the 5-HT$_{2A}$, 5-HT$_{2C}$ and GABA$_{A\alpha6}$ receptors and the serotonin transporter in the level of response to alcohol: a pilot study. *Biol Psychiatry.* **45**(5): 647–51.

Seale JP (1991) *Confronting Barriers to Substance Abuse: diagnosis and treatment in project SAEFP workshop, substance abuse education for family physicians.* The Society of Teachers of Family Medicine, Kansas City, MO.

Seitz HK, Simanowski UA, Egerer G, Waldherr R and Oertl U (1992) Human gastric alcohol dehydrogenase: *in vitro* characteristics and effects of cimetidine. *Digestion.* **51**(2): 80–5.

Selzer M (1971) The Michigan Alcoholism Screening Test (MAST): validation of a new alcoholism screening instrument. *Am J Psychiatry.* **127**: 1653–8.

Selzer M (1971) Michigan Alcoholism Screening Test: the quest for a new diagnostic instrument. *Am J Psychiatry.* **127**: 89–94.

Selzer M, Vinokur A and Van Rooijan L (1975) A self-administered short Michigan Alcoholism Screening Test (SMAST). *J Stud Alcohol.* **36**: 117–26.

Sher K (1994) Individual-level risk factors. In: R Zucker, G Boyd and J Howard (eds) *The Development of Alcohol Problems: exploring the bio-psycho-social matrix of risk.* National Institute on Alcohol Abuse and Alcoholism, Rockville, MD.

Silk-Walker P, Walter D and Kivlahan D (1988) Alcoholism, alcohol abuse and health in American Indians and Alaskan Natives. In: S Manson and N Dinges (eds) *Behavioral Health Issues Among American Indians and Alaskan Natives: explorations on the frontiers of the biobehavioral sciences.* National Center for American Indian and Alaskan Native Mental Health Research, Denver, CO.

Simmons GM (1991) *Interpersonal trust and perceived locus of control in the adjustment of adult children of alcoholics* (dissertation), US International University, San Diego, CA. Unpublished.

Single E (1994) Implications of potential health benefits of moderate drinking for specific elements of alcohol policy: towards a harm reduction approach for alcohol. *Contemp Drug Probl.* **21**: 273–85.

Sisson RW and Mallams JH (1981) Use of systematic encouragement and community access procedures to increase attendance at Alcoholics Anonymous and Al-Anon meetings. *Am J Drug Alcohol Abuse.* **8**(3): 371–6.

Sokol RJ, Ager J, Martier S *et al.* (1986) Significant determinants of susceptibility to alcohol teratogenicity. *Ann NY Acad Sci.* **477**: 87–102.

Steffian G (1999) Correction of normative misperceptions: an alcohol abuse prevention program. *J Drug Educ.* **29**(2): 115–38.

Steinbauer JR, Cantor SB, Holzer CE and Volk RJ (1998) Ethnic and sex bias in primary care screening tests for alcohol use disorders. *Ann Intern Med.* **129**: 353–62.

Steinglass P, Davis D and Berenson D (1977) Observations of conjointly hospitalized 'alcoholic couples' during sobriety and intoxication: implications for theory and therapy. *Fam Process.* **16**(1): 1–16.

Steinglass P, Bennett L, Wolin S and Reiss D (1987) *The Alcoholic Family.* Basic Books, New York.

Steinweg DL and Worth H (1993) Alcoholism: the key to the CAGE. *Am J Med.* **94**: 520–3.

Stephens GG (1982) *The Intellectual Basis of Family Practice.* Winter Publishing, Tuscon, AZ.

Stewart J and Vezina P (1988) A comparison of the effects of intra-accumbens injections of amphetamine and morphine on re-instatement of heroin intravenous self-administration behavior. *Brain Res.* **457**: 287–94.

Stewart M (2001) Towards a global definition of patient-centred care. *BMJ.* **322**(7284): 444–5.

Stewart M, Brown JB, Weston W *et al.* (1995) *Patient-Centered Medicine: transforming the clinical method.* Sage Publications Inc, Thousand Oaks, CA.

Strunin L and Hingson R (1992) Alcohol, drugs and adolescent sexual behavior. *Int J Addict.* **27**(2): 129–46.

Swenson WM and Morse RM (1975) The use of a self-administered alcoholism screening test (SAAST). *Mayo Clin Proc.* **50**: 204–8.

Tabakoff B, Hoffman PL, Lee JM *et al.* (1988) Differences in platelet enzyme activity between alcoholics and controls. *NEJM.* **318**: 134–9.

Taj N, Devera-Sales A and Vinso DC (1998) Screening for problem drinking: does a single question work? *J Fam Pract.* **46**(4): 328–35.

US Bureau of the Census (1991) *Current Populations Reports: Series P-20, No. 449.* US Government Printing Office, USBC, Washington, DC.

US Bureau of the Census (1992) *Statistical Abstract of the US: 1992* (112e). US Government Printing Office, USBC, Washington, DC.

US Census Bureau (1998) *The Official Statistical Abstract of the US: 1998* (118e). US Department of Commerce, USBC, Washington, DC.

US Department of Health and Human Services, Public Health Service, Alcohol, Drug Abuse, and Mental Health Administration, National Institute on Alcohol Abuse and Alcoholism

(1990) *Seventh Special Report to the US Congress on Alcohol and Health*. US Government Printing Office, USDHHS, Washington, DC.

US Department of Health and Human Services (1991) *Health Status of Minorities and Low Income Groups* (3e). US Government Printing Office, USDHHS, Washington, DC.

US Department of Health and Human Services, Public Health Service, National Institutes of Health, National Institute on Alcohol Abuse and Alcoholism (1993) *Eighth Special Report to the US Congress on Alcohol and Health*. US Government Printing Office, USDHHS, Washington, DC.

US Department of Health and Human Services, Public Health Service, National Institutes of Health, National Institute on Alcohol Abuse and Alcoholism (1997) *Ninth Special Report to the US Congress on Alcohol and Health*. US Government Printing Office, USDHHS, Washington, DC.

US Department of Health and Human Services, Office of Applied Studies, Substance Abuse and Mental Health Services Administration (1998) *National Household Survey on Drug Abuse: main findings 1996*. US Government Printing Office, USDHHS, Washington, DC.

Vaillant GE (1995) *The Natural History of Alcoholism Revisited*. Harvard University Press, Cambridge, MA.

Vaillant GE (1996) A long-term follow-up of male alcohol abuse. *Arch Gen Psychiatry*. **53**: 243–9.

Vaillant GE and Blumenthal SJ (1990) Introduction: Suicide over the lifecycle: risk factors and life-span development. In: SJ Blumenthal and DJ Kupfer (eds) *Suicide over the Lifecycle: risk factors, assessment, and treatment of suicidal patients*. American Psychiatric Press, Washington, DC.

Vestal RE, McGuire EA, Tobin JD *et al.* (1977) Aging and alcohol metabolism. *Clin Pharmacol Ther*. **21**: 343–54.

Volavka J, Czobor P, Goodwin DW *et al.* (1996) The electroencephalogram after alcohol administration in high-risk men and the development of alcohol use disorders 10 years later. *Arch Gen Psychiatry*. **53**: 258–63.

Volk RJ, Cantor SB, Steinbauer JR and Cass AR (1997) Item bias in the CAGE screening test for alcohol use disorders. *J Gen Intern Med*. **12**: 763–9.

Volkow ND *et al.* (1993) Decreased dopamine D2 receptor availability is associated with reduced frontal metabolism in cocaine abusers. *Synapse*. **14**(2): 169–77.

Volpicelli JR, Alterman A, Hayashida M and O'Brien CP (1992) Naltrexone in the treatment of alcohol dependence. *Arch Gen Psychiatry*. **49**(11): 876–80.

Volpicelli JR, Watson NT, King AC *et al.* (1995) Effect of naltrexone on alcohol 'high' in alcoholics. *Am J Psychiatry*. **152**(4): 613–15.

Waller MB, McBride WJ, Gatto GJ *et al.* (1984) Intragastric self-infusion of ethanol by ethanol-preferring and non-preferring lines of rats. *Science*. **225**: 78–80.

Wegscheider S (1981) *Another Chance: hope and health for the alcoholic family*. Science and Behavior Books, Palo Alto, CA.

Weibel-Orlando J (1985) *IHS, Alcohol Abuse and Future Research Directions: Review of the Indian Health Service Alcoholism Program*. US Government Printing Office, Denver, CO.

Weibel-Orlando JC, Weisner T and Long J (1984) Urban and rural Indian drinking patterns: implications for intervention and policy development. *Subst Alcohol Actions/Misuse*. **5**: 45–57.

Weingardt KR and Marlatt GA (1998) Sustaining change: helping those who are still using. In: W Miller and N Heather (eds) *Treating Addictive Behaviors* (2e). Plenum, New York.

Weizmann D (ed.) (2000) *Drinking with Bukowski: recollections of the Poet Laureate of Skid Row*. Thunder's Mouth Press, New York.

Westermeyer J (1976) Use of a social indicator system to assess alcoholism among Indian people in Minnesota. *Am J Drug Alcohol Abuse*. **3**(3): 447–56.

Westermeyer J (1979) 'The drunken Indian': myths and realities. In: M Marshall (ed.) *Beliefs, Behaviors and Alcoholic Beverages: a cross-cultural survey*. University of Michigan Press, Ann Arbor, MI.

Westermeyer J (1982) Alcoholism and services for ethnic populations. In: E Pattison and E Kaufman (eds) *Encyclopedic Handbook of Alcoholism*. Gardner Press Inc, New York.

Westermeyer JJ and Baker JM (1986) Alcoholism and the American Indian. In: NJ Estes and ME Heinemann (eds) *Alcoholism: development, consequences and interventions* (3e). Mosby, St Louis, MO.

Weston WW, Brown JB and Stewart MA (1989) Patient-centred interviewing Part I: understanding patients' experiences. *Can Fam Physician*. **35**: 147–51.

Whitcup SM and Miller F (1987) Unrecognized drug dependence in psychiatrically hospitalized elderly patients. *J Am Geriatr Soc*. **35**: 297–301.

White WL (2000) The role of recovering physicians in 19th century addiction medicine: an organizational case study. *J Addict Dis*. **19**(2): 1–10.

Williams TP and Lillis RP (1988) Long-term changes in reported alcohol purchasing and consumption following an increase in New York State's purchase age to 19. *Br J Addict*. **83**(2): 209–17.

Wilsnack SC (1996) Patterns and trends in women's drinking: recent findings and some implications for prevention. In: JM Howard, SE Martin, PD Mail *et al.* (eds) *Women and Alcohol: issues for prevention research*. NIAAA Research Monograph No. 32. US Department of Health and Human Services, Bethesda, MD.

Wilsnack SC and Wilsnack RW (1995) Drinking and problem drinking among US women: patterns and recent trends. In: M Galanter (ed.) *Recent Developments in Alcoholism. Volume 12: alcoholism and women: the effect of gender*. Plenum, New York.

Wilsnack SC, Klassen AD, Schur BE and Wilsnack RW (1991) Predicting onset and chronicity of women's problem drinking: a 5-year longitudinal analysis. *Am J Pub Health*. **81**(3): 305–18.

Wilsnack SC, Wilsnack RW and Hiller-Sturmhopel S (1994) How women drink: epidemiology of women's drinking and problem drinking. *Alcohol Health Res World*. **18**(3): 173–81.

Wolin SJ and Wolin S (1993) *The Resilient Self: how survivors of troubled families rise above adversity.* Villard Books, New York.

Wolin S, Bennett L and Noonan D (1979) Family rituals and the recurrence of alcoholism over generations. *Am J Psychiatry.* **136**(4B): 589–93.

Wolin S, Bennett L, Noonan D and Teitelbaum M (1980) Disrupted family rituals: a factor in the intergenerational transmission of alcoholism. *J Stud Alcohol.* **41**(3): 199–214.

Yersin B, Nicolet JF, Decrey H *et al.* (1995) Screening for excessive alcohol drinking: comparative value of carbohydrate-deficient transferrin, gamma-glutamyltransferase and mean corpuscular volume. *Arch Intern Med.* **155**(17): 1907–11.

Zimberg S (1995) The elderly. In: AM Washton (ed.) *Psychotherapy and Substance Abuse: a practitioner's guide.* Guilford Press, New York.

Zimberg S, Wallace J and Blume S (1985) *Practical Approaches to Alcoholism Psychotherapy* (2e). Plenum, New York.

Zimberg S, Wallace J and Blume S (1987) *Practical Approaches to Alcoholism in Psychotherapy* (2e). Plenum, New York.

Zucker R (1994) Pathways to alcohol problems and alcoholism: a developmental account of the evidence for multiple alcoholisms and for contextual contributions to risk. In: R Zucker, G Boyd and J Howard (eds) *The Development of Alcohol Problems: exploring the bio-psycho-social matrix of risk.* National Institute on Alcohol Abuse and Alcoholism, Rockville, MD.

Index